Weight Watchers
Freestyle Air Fryer Cookbook 2020

Healthy & Delicious WW Smart Points Recipes for Your Air Fryer to Live Happier and Feel Better

By
Sam Cook

Copyright © **Sam Cook** 2019

All rights reserved. No part of this publication maybe reproduced, stored or
transmitted in any form or by any means, electronic, mechanical, photocopying,
recording, scanning, or otherwise without written permission from the author. It is
illegal to copy this book, post it to a website, or distribute it by any other means
without permission.

Sam Cook the moral right to be identified as the author of this work.

TABLE OF CONTENTS

INTRODUCTION 8
What is Weight Watchers 9
WW Airfryer Breakfast Recipes 11
   Air Fryer 2 Ingredient Weight Watcher Friendly Bagels .. 11
   Air Fryer Egg Souffle is Weight Watchers Friendly! 12
   Air Fryer Breakfast Bake 13
   Air Fryer French Toast Sticks 14
   Air Fryer Breakfast Burritos 15
   Air Fryer-Perfectly Done, Heavenly French Toast 16
   Cheesy Breakfast Egg Rolls 17
   Air Fryer Breakfast Frittata 18
   Air Fryer Scotch Eggs 21
   Air Fryer Roasted Potatoes 23
   Air Fryer Bacon and Egg Breakfast Biscuit Bombs 24
   Breakfast Air Fried Potatoes 25
   Air Fryer Breakfast Flautas 27
   Easy Air Fryer Omelette 28
   Air Fryer Egg Rolls 30
WW Airfryer Vegetarian Recipes 32
   Cheese and Veggie Egg Cups 32
   Air Fryer Brussel Sprouts 33
   Air Fried Tofu Italian Style 33
   Vegan Air Fryer Buffalo Cauliflower 35

Air Fryer Roasted Cauliflower 36

Air Fryer Chickpeas 37

Air Fryer Buffalo Cauliflower 38

Get Crispy Veggie Quesadillas in an Air Fryer 40

Air-Fryer Vegan French "Toast" 41

Air Fryer Brussel Sprouts (Extra Crispy!) 42

Air Fryer Vegetable Kebabs 43

Air Fryer Broccoli Parmesan 44

Blackened Air Fryer Salmon with Cucumber-Avocado Salsa 45

Vegan Air Fryer Buffalo Cauliflower 47

Air-Fried Vegan Tofu 48

WW Airfryer Fish & Seafood Recipes 50

Weight Watcher Oven Fried Fish 50

Healthy Baked Fish Sticks with Lemon Caper Sauce 51

Air Fryer Tuna Cakes Recipe 52

Air-Fried Crumbed Fish 53

PointsPlus "Fried" Catfish with Potato Sticks Recipe 54

Soy-Glazed Fish with Stir-Fried Spinach 55

Air Fryer Fish and Chips Healthy 56

Extra Crispy Air Fryer Bacon Recipe 57

Air Fryer Fish 57

Air Fryer garlic lime shrimp kabobs 59

Air Fryer Parmesan Shrimp 59

Air Fryer Weight Watchers Crab Wontons 60

Easy Baked Tilapia 62

Cilantro Lime Air Fryer Shrimp Skewers 63

Air Fryer Bang Bang Shrimp (with lightened up sauce) .. 64

Low Fat Parmesan Crusted Tilapia 66

Oven Fried Shrimp Recipe (5 WW points) 67

Air Fryer Shrimp Egg Rolls 69

Low Carb Meatballs in the Airfryer 70

Air Fryer Fish And Chips 71

WW Airfryer Poultry Recipes 72

Buffalo Style Air Fryer Chicken Wings 72

Air Fryer Chicken Nuggets 73

Air Fryer Whole Chicken 75

Crispy Air Fryer Chicken Breast 77

Air Fryer Greek Stuffed Chicken Breast 78

The Best Air Fryer Popcorn Chicken 79

Air Fryer Chicken Milanese with Arugula 80

Air Fryer Asian-Glazed Boneless Chicken Thighs 82

Chicken Parmesan in the Air Fryer 83

Air-Fryer Chicken Potstickers 84

Quick Air Fryer Tortilla Chips 85

Air Fryer Buffalo Chicken Tenders 86

FireCracker Chicken, Slimming & W W Friendly 87

Cornflake chicken 89

Air Fryer Chick-fil-A Chicken Sandwich 89

Air Fryer Greek Stuffed Chicken Breast 92

Chicken schnitzel with salsa verde 93

Air Fried Chicken Philly Cheese Egg Rolls 95

Crispy Air Fryer Chicken Tenders... 96

Air Fryer Chicken Tenders... 97

WW Airfryer Beef & Pork Recipes 99

Air Fryer Beef Empanadas 100

That Man's Pork Chops 101

Beef and Vegetables Stir Fry with Noodles 102

Beef and Broccoli Stir-Fry.. 103

Ww Oven-Fried Pork Chops 5-Points 104

Barbecued Pork Chops 105

Pork Cacciatore... 106

Air-fried Burgers 108

Crispy Breaded Pork Chops in the Air Fryer 109

WW Airfryer Soups and Stews Recipes..................................111

Healthy & Quick W W Instant Pot Chicken Noodle Soup
.... 111

Weight Watchers Zero Point Asian Soup Recipe 112

Greek Orzo and Chicken Soup.. 113

Whole Wheat Orzo, Cauliflower & Kale Soup.................. 114

Spaghetti & Meatball Soup 115

Smoked Ham Soup with White Beans 117

Italian Vegetable Soup... 118

Chicken Vegetable Soup Recipe... 120

Zucchini and Rosemary Soup.. 121

Slow Cooker Potato Soup for Weight Watchers 122

WW Airfryer Desserts Recipes 123
   Air Fryer Baked Potato Recipe - Baked Garlic Parsley Potatoes
   123
   Air Fryer Chickpea Tacos 124
   2 Ingredient Dough Cinnamon Rolls 125
   Air Fryer Monkey Bread 126
   Weight Watchers Air Fryer Empanadas 127
   Air Fryer Pork Taquitos 128
   Air Fryer Chimichangas 129
   Weight Watchers Donuts 130
   Air Fryer Funnel Cake Bites 131
   Air Fryer Tuna Cakes Recipe 132
CONCLUSION 133

INTRODUCTION

Anyone who has ever even thought about dieting has undoubtedly heard of the Weight Watchers plan. It is one of the most common weight loss programs out there, and offers not only weight loss products and weight loss supplements, but has a unique system of meetings and support that few diet plans offer.

But just why has Weight Watchers become so successful and why does the company continue to expand after more than 45 years in operation?

The answer lies in the fact that Weight Watchers does not simply offer a diet plan but is based upon the philosophy of dieting as part of an overall plan to set and maintain a healthy lifestyle in terms of physical, mental and emotional health.

Consequently, Weight Watchers does not just provide you with a diet sheet and tell you what you can and can't eat, but provides you with the information and advice necessary to make the best decisions about your diet.

Further, and very importantly, the Weight Watchers plan gives you a level of support and motivation that is essential to your success and that is lacking in so many other weight loss plans.

WHAT IS WEIGHT WATCHERS

Weight Watchers is a diet and healthy eating program characterized by its now famous point system, which assigns meals and foods a certain number of points. Each meal is given a different point number based on its total caloric value, how much fat is in the meal, how many carbohydrates are in the meal, and various other nutritional values. Separate foods are also given point values. When following a Weight Watcher's meal plan, a person has a certain ideal point range for each day, and the goal is to stay under or within that particular range in order to lose weight.

Because the WW program relies heavily on its unique point system, many followers of the program use Weight Watchers recipes to ensure that they know the exact points of the meals and food they eat. Thankfully, the company provides its customers with a wide variety of recipes. Some people might be wary of a recipe book based on the unique point system, thinking that they will be restricted to a few types of meals; however, there are hundreds of hundreds of official recipes available to followers of the WW program. And that's not including any of the custom, homemade recipes created by WW followers!

There are so many different recipes to find in WW books, pamphlets, and online material. Each recipe comes with a set of instructions, a list of ingredients, and the number of points that each serving of the recipe will contain. Weight Watchers recipes are notoriously varied and generally easy enough for any home cooker to make! The recipes aren't limited to typical diet fare like salads, fruits, and vegetables, or other low-fat meals, either! The clientele for Weight Watchers is so diverse that they have created recipes for just about any food taste! Dinner when following one of the program's recipes could be fajitas, typical hamburgers, or a fancy gumbo! Dessert could be as simple as fresh watermelon and yogurt, or a deliciously rich chocolate fondue dip. The program doesn't limit dieters to bland or boring foods, and with the easy point system, it's simple to make sure that one stays within their appointed point range.

One of the most popular features of Weight Watchers recipes are their low point value, healthy nutrition, and fulfilling portions. These three attributes combined lead to a diverse diet that improves the health of those that follow the recipes and point system. Some diet programs might have dieters fill up on cheap preservatives and carbohydrates in order to trick them into thinking that they are full and eating a good amount of food., when in fact they are simply filling up on starch, which can be unhealthy in large amounts. Weight Watchers, however, seeks to not only help people control how much food they eat, but what kinds of food they are eating. Food made from Weight Watchers recipes will be both healthy, delicious, filling, and help the dieter lose weight and control their appetite.

WW AIRFRYER BREAKFAST RECIPES

Air Fryer 2 Ingredient Weight Watcher Friendly Bagels

Prep/Cook Time: 15 minutes, Servings : 4 , 3 WW Freestyle Smartpoint

Ingredients

- 1 cup self rising flour
- 1 cup low greek yogurt
- 1 egg

Instructions

- Mix together yogurt and flour until becomes a ball of dough.
- Place ball of dough on a flat dry surface and cover with flour.
- Separate into 4 balls.
- Roll each ball into a long rope
- Shape into a bagel form.
- Whisk egg.
- Coat each bagel with an egg wash and any toppings.
- Place in air fryer or ninja basket
- Place on 350 for 10 minutes.

Nutrition Info : Calories: 162 Total Fat: 2g Saturated Fat: 1g Trans Fat: 0g Unsaturated Fat: 1g Cholesterol: 49mg Sodium: 411mg Carbohydrates: 25g Fiber: 1g Sugar: 2g Protein: 10g

Air Fryer Egg Souffle is Weight Watchers Friendly!

Prep/Cook Time, 4 servings, 0 WW Freestyle Smartpoint

Ingredients

- 4 large Eggs
- 1/2 cup mushrooms
- 1/2 cup broccoli florets
- 1 spray cooking spray (a few)
- 1 tsp crushed red pepper
- 1 tsp garlic powder
- 1 tsp minced onions (use onion powder if you like :))

Instructions

- Spray ramekins with pan spray
- In a medium sized bowl scramble eggs, garlic, onion and red pepper together.
- Add broccoli and mushrooms mix well
- Pour eggs into ramekins
- Place ramekins into the airfryer
- 350 for 15 minutes, make sure the eggs are cooked. If not, air fry for another 5 minutes.
- Serve hot

Nutrition Info : Calories: 200 Total Fat: 2.3g Saturated Fat: 3g, Carbohydrates: 16g Fiber: 2g Sugar: 2g Protein: 13g

Air Fryer Breakfast Bake

Prep/Cook Time: 45mins, SERVES: 2, 4 WW Freestyle Smartpoint

Ingredients

- 4 eggs
- 2 tablespoons 1% low-fat milk
- 1/2 teaspoon kosher salt
- 1 teaspoon hot sauce
- 1 slice whole grain bread, torn into pieces
- 1 1/2 cups Baby Spinach
- 1/4 cup shredded cheddar cheese
- 1/2 cup diced bell pepper
- 2 tablespoons shredded cheddar cheese

Instructions

- Preheat air fryer to 250-degrees F. Spray a 6-inch soufflé dish with nonstick cooking spray; set aside.
- Beat eggs, milk, salt and hot sauce in a medium bowl.
- Fold in bread pieces, spinach, ¼ cup cheese and bell pepper.
- Pour egg mixture into prepared casserole dish and transfer dish to the air fryer basket.
- Cook for 20 minutes. Pause the machine, sprinkle with remaining cheese and cook for an additional 5 minutes or until eggs are completely set and the edges are golden brown.
- Carefully remove from fryer basket and allow to rest for 10 minutes before serving.

Nutrition Info : Calories: 165; Total Fat: 9 grams; Saturated Fat: 4 grams; Total Carbohydrate: 14 grams; Sugars: 2 grams; Protein: 9 grams

Air Fryer French Toast Sticks

Prep/Cook Time: 15 minutes, 2 Servings, 3 WW Freestyle Smartpoint

Ingredients

- 2 slices of gluten-free, whole grain, or sprouted grain bread…find something that is hearty and not too soft.
- 1 egg
- 3T unsweetened vanilla almond milk or whatever milk you have
- 2tsp maple syrup, plus more for dipping
- 1/2 tsp cinnamon or more
- ½ tsp pure vanilla extract
- cooking oil spray (I used coconut oil spray)

Instructions

- Line bottom of air fryer basket with parchment paper – this is super important, as it prevents sticking.
- Next, slice your bread into 4 equal sticks. Mix egg, milk, maple syrup, vanilla and cinnamon together. Dip bread into egg mixture and coat well, but shake off the excess egg.
- Place sticks on parchment and spray with cooking oil spray. Don't overcrowd them – you may need to do two batches if your Air Fryer is really small.
- Set to 360 and cook for ten minutes, flipping halfway and removing the parchment paper for the second half of cooking. You may need a little more or a little less time depending on your desired crispiness. We liked ours very crispy!

Nutrition Info : Calories: 150; Total Fat: 11 grams; Saturated Fat: 4 grams; Total Carbohydrate: 45grams; Sugars: 2 grams; Protein: 7 grams

Air Fryer Breakfast Burritos

Prep/Cook Time: 23 minutes, Servings: 8, 5 WW Freestyle Smartpoint

Ingredients

- 1 pound breakfast sausage
- 1 bell pepper, chopped
- 12 eggs beaten together
- 1/2 teaspoon black pepper
- 1 teaspoon sea salt
- 8 flour tortillas burrito size
- 2 cups shredded colby jack cheese or use your favorite cheese

Instructions

- Crumble and cook the sausage in a large skillet until brown. Stir in chopped peppers. Drain grease, place sausage on paper towel-lined plate, cover and set aside
- In a large skillet, melt 1 tablespoon of butter, add eggs, salt and pepper, and cook over medium heat, stirring continuously, until mostly set and no longer runny
- Stir in cooked sausage, then remove from heat
- Add some of the egg and sausage mixture to the middle of a tortilla, top with some of the cheese, fold sides, and roll up
- Preheat air fryer to 390 degrees
- Spray burritos lightly with olive oil spray
- Place as many burritos as will fit into the air fryer or Instant Pot Vortex trays, and cook for 3 minutes at 390 degrees for basket air fryers and 2 minutes in the

Vortex, rotating trays halfway through. For extra dark or crispier burritos, cook for 3 minutes in the Vortex
- Remove and serve immediately, or allow to cool slightly, then wrap well and freeze for meal prep

Nutrition Info : Calories: 283kcal, Carbohydrates: 16g, Protein: 16g, Fat: 17g, Saturated Fat: 8g, Cholesterol: 234mg, Sodium: 750mg

Air Fryer-Perfectly Done, Heavenly French Toast

Prep/Cook Time: 20 mins, Servings: 4, 4 WW Freestyle Smartpoint

Ingredients

- 4 slices of bread
- 2 eggs
- 1/4 cup of milk
- 1 teaspoon of vanilla
- 1 tablespoon of cinnamon

Instructions

- In a small bowl mix together the eggs, milk, cinnamon, and vanilla. Then beat until the eggs are broken up and everything is mixed well.
- Then dip each piece of bread into the mixture and then shake to get the excess off, as you do, put them into your prepared pan
- Air Fryer for 3 minutes at 320 degrees F. Then flip them over and do another 3 minutes.
- Serve with maple syrup and enjoy!

Nutrition Info : Calories: 263kcal, Carbohydrates: 22g, Protein: 15g, Fat: 16g, Saturated Fat: 8g, Cholesterol: 134mg, Sodium: 500mg

Cheesy Breakfast Egg Rolls

Prep/Cook Time:Prep: 40 min./batch, 12 servings, 3 WW Freestyle Smartpoint

Ingredients

- 1/2 pound bulk pork sausage
- 1/2 cup shredded sharp cheddar cheese
- 1/2 cup shredded Monterey Jack cheese
- 1 tablespoon chopped green onions
- 4 large eggs
- 1 tablespoon 2% milk
- 1/4 teaspoon salt
- 1/8 teaspoon pepper
- 1 tablespoon butter
- 12 egg roll wrappers
- Maple syrup or salsa, optional

Instructions

- In a small nonstick skillet, cook sausage over medium heat until no longer pink, 4-6 minutes, breaking into crumbles; drain. Stir in cheeses and green onions; set aside. Wipe skillet clean.
- In a small bowl, whisk eggs, milk, salt and pepper until blended. In the same skillet, heat butter over medium heat. Pour in egg mixture; cook and stir until eggs are thickened and no liquid egg remains. Stir in sausage mixture.
- Preheat air fryer to 400°. With one corner of an egg roll wrapper facing you, place 1/4 cup filling just below center of wrapper. (Cover remaining wrappers with a

damp paper towel until ready to use.) Fold bottom corner over filling; moisten remaining wrapper edges with water. Fold side corners toward center over filling. Roll egg roll up tightly, pressing at tip to seal. Repeat.
- o In batches, arrange egg rolls in a single layer in greased air-fryer basket; spritz with cooking spray. Cook until lightly browned, 3-4 minutes. Turn; spritz with cooking spray. Cook until golden brown and crisp, 3-4 minutes longer. If desired, serve with maple syrup or salsa.

Nutrition Info : 209 calories, 10g fat (4g saturated fat), 87mg cholesterol, 438mg sodium, 19g carbohydrate (0 sugars, 1g fiber), 10g protein.

Air Fryer Breakfast Frittata

Prep/Cook Time: 20 mins, Servings: 4, 3 WW Freestyle Smartpoint

Ingredients

Breakfast Frittata Ingredients:

- 4 eggs
- 3 tablespoons heavy cream double cream
- 4 tablespoons grated cheddar cheese
- 4 mushrooms sliced
- 3 grape tomatoes cherry tomatoes, halved
- 4 tablespoons chopped spinach
- 2 tablespoons fresh chopped herbs of choice
- 1 green onion sliced

- salt to taste

Instructions

Air Fryer Frittata Recipe Instructions:

- Preheat the air fryer to 350 F / 180 C.
- Line a deep 7-inch baking pan with parchment paper, then oil the pan and set it aside.
- In a bowl, whisk together the eggs and cream.
- Add the rest of the ingredients to the bowl, and stir to combine.
- Pour the breakfast frittata mixture into the baking pan and place inside the air fryer basket.
- Cook for 12-16 minutes, or until eggs are set. To check, insert a toothpick in the center of the air fryer frittata. The eggs are set if it comes out clean.

Air Fryer Breakfast Frittata Tips

- As the eggs can stick to the pan, lining it with parchment and then oiling it is important.
- Feel free to vary the veggies in this recipe to suit your taste. Just make sure to stick with quick cooking veggies.
- This breakfast frittata is a great way to use up any leftover meat you might have. Toss in some diced ham, shredded chicken, or crumbled bacon. Yum!

Nutrition Info : Serving: 2g, Calories: 147kcal, Carbohydrates: 3g, Protein: 9g, Fat: 11g, Saturated Fat: 6g, Cholesterol: 188mg, Sodium: 133mg, Potassium: 237mg, Fiber: 1g, Sugar: 1g

Air Fryer Scotch Eggs

Scotch eggs, a classic pub snack, gets a modern upgrade in this panko-coated air

Prep/Cook Time: 45 mins, Servings: 64 WW Freestyle Smartpoin

Ingredients

- 1/2 cup finely chopped onion
- 1 tablespoon snipped fresh chives
- 2 cloves garlic, minced
- 1 teaspoon snipped fresh thyme
- 1 teaspoon salt
- 1 teaspoon pepper
- ½ teaspoon snipped fresh sage
- 1 pound ground pork
- ½ cup all-purpose flour
- ½ teaspoon smoked paprika (optional)
- 2 eggs
- 2 tablespoons water
- 1½ cups panko bread crumbs
- 6 eggs, hard-cooked or soft-boiled, peeled*
- ½ cup mayonnaise
- 1 – 2 tablespoon Sriracha sauce
- 2 teaspoons lemon juice
- 6 cups arugula or fresh spinach

Instructions

- Preheat airfryer to 350°F. In a medium bowl combine onion, chives, 1 clove garlic, thyme, 1/2 tsp. salt, 1/2 tsp pepper, and sage. Add ground pork; mix well.
- In a shallow dish combine flour, remaining 1/2 tsp. salt and pepper, and paprika, if using. In another shallow

dish beat together 2 eggs and water. In another shallow dish place panko.
- Dip each cooked egg in the flour mixture. Divide meat mixture into six portions. Flatten into thin patties and fold around hard cooked eggs, sealing and smoothing edges to completely enclose.
- Working gently with 1 sausage-wrapped egg at a time, dip eggs again into flour, shaking off excess, then coat in lightly beaten eggs. Roll in panko to coat.
- Place scotch eggs in airfryer basket (do not overcrowd). Cook eggs 15 minutes or until golden brown.
- Meanwhile, in a small bowl combine mayonnaise, Sriracha, lemon juice, and remaining 1 clove garlic. Serve eggs warm over arugula and drizzle with spicy mayonnaise.

Tips

- For hard-cooked eggs, place eggs in a single layer in a large saucepan. Add cold water to cover by 1-inch. Bring to a full rolling boil. Remove from heat, cover and let stand for 15 minutes. Drain; place in ice water until cool enough to handle. Peel eggs. For soft-boiled eggs, bring water to boiling. Using a slotted spoon, gently lower eggs into water. Reduce heat to maintain a gentle boil.
- Boil 6 minutes for soft boiled or 8 minutes for a jammy but not set yolk. Drain; place in ice water until cool enough to handle. Peel eggs. If using soft-boiled eggs, use a gentle hand when enclosing them in the meat mixture.

Nutrition Info : 426 calories, (8 g saturated fat, 11 g polyunsaturated fat, 11 g monounsaturated fat), 277 mg cholesterol, 725 mg sodium, 10 g carbohydrates, 1 g fiber, 2 g sugar, 23 g protein.

Air Fryer Roasted Potatoes

Air fryer roasted potatoes with garlic and herbs are cooked to golden, crispy perfection. They are the perfect side dish for breakfast, lunch or dinner.

Prep/Cook Time: 27 minutes, Servings 4, 4 WW Freestyle Smartpoint

Ingredients

- 1.5 pounds potatoes (diced into 1 inch pieces - gold, red or russets)
- 1/2 teaspoon garlic powder or granulated garlic
- 1/2 teaspoon salt or more, to taste
- 1/4 teaspoon pepper
- 1/2 teaspoon oregano dried
- 1/2 teaspoon basil dried
- cooking spray (I am using avocado oil cooking spray)

Instructions

- Spray the air fryer cooking basket with the cooking spray.
- Add diced potatoes to the basket, and give the potatoes a spray.
- Add salt, pepper, garlic powder, oregano and basil, and toss to combine and evenly coat the potatoes.
- Cook at 400 degrees (not preheated) until brown and crispy, about 20 to 24 minutes.
- Toss them half way through with a flipper, and shake the basket once more to ensure even cooking.

Nutrition Info : Calories 110 Calories from Fat 9, Fat 1g, Sodium 308mg, Potassium 702mg, Carbohydrates 21g, Fiber 4g, Protein 4g

Air Fryer Bacon and Egg Breakfast Biscuit Bombs

Prep/Cook Time: 50 min, Servings 8, 4 WW Freestyle Smartpoint

Ingredients
- Biscuit Bombs
- 4 slices bacon, cut into 1/2-inch pieces
- 1 tablespoon butter
- 2 eggs, beaten
- 1/4 teaspoon pepper
- 1 can (10.2 oz) Pillsbury™ Grands!™ Southern Homestyle refrigerated Buttermilk biscuits (5 biscuits)
- 2 oz sharp cheddar cheese, cut into ten 3/4-inch cubes
- Egg Wash
- 1 egg
- 1 tablespoon water

Instructions

- Cut two 8-inch rounds of cooking parchment paper. Place one round in bottom of air fryer basket. Spray with cooking spray.
- In 10-inch nonstick skillet, cook bacon over medium-high heat until crisp. Remove from pan; place on paper towel. Carefully wipe skillet with paper towel. Add butter to skillet; melt over medium heat. Add 2 beaten eggs and pepper to skillet; cook until eggs are

- thickened but still moist, stirring frequently. Remove from heat; stir in bacon. Cool 5 minutes.
  o Meanwhile, separate dough into 5 biscuits; separate each biscuit into 2 layers. Press each into 4-inch round. Spoon 1 heaping tablespoonful egg mixture onto center of each round. Top with one piece of the cheese. Gently fold edges up and over filling; pinch to seal. In small bowl, beat remaining egg and water. Brush biscuits on all sides with egg wash.
  o Place 5 of the biscuit bombs, seam sides down, on parchment in air fryer basket. Spray both sides of second parchment round with cooking spray. Top biscuit bombs in basket with second parchment round, then top with remaining 5 biscuit bombs.
  o Set to 325°F; cook 8 minutes. Remove top parchment round; using tongs, carefully turn biscuits, and place in basket in single layer. Cook 4 to 6 minutes longer or until cooked through (at least 165°F).

Nutrition Info : Calories 200, Calories from Fat 100, Total Fat 12g, Saturated Fat 6g, Protein 7g

Breakfast Air Fried Potatoes

Prep/Cook Time: 1 hour 10 mins, Servings 2, 5 WW Freestyle Smartpoint

Ingredients

- 2 medium Russet Potatoes
- 1/2 tsp salt
- 1 Tbsp olive oil

- 1/4 tsp garlic powder
- chopped parsley for garnish

Instructions

- Clean and scrub potatoes under running water. Dice potatoes into 1/2 inch cubes.
- Place potatoes in bowl and cover with ice cold water. Allow to soak for 45 minutes.
- Remove potatoes from water and dry with paper towels. Add potatoes in dry bowl and add olive oil, salt, garlic powder. Stir potatoes ensuring that all pieces are covered in oil.
- Place in air fryer basket. Cook at 400 degrees Farenheit 20-23 minutes, shaking the basket halfway through. Potatoes are done when they are golden brown on the outside and soft on the inside.
- Top with parsley if desired.

Notes on Breakfast Air Fried Potatoes

- You can do more or less potatoes in the Air Fryer. Cook time will remain the same, just ensure to shake halfway through.
- Careful not to overcrowd the air fryer basket. A single layer of potatoes is ideal but some overlap is ok. Shake basket to ensure even cooking.

Nutrition Info : Calories: 170kcal, Fat 2g, Sodium 200mg, Potassium 640mg, Carbohydrates 21g, Fiber 04g, Protein 4g

Air Fryer Breakfast Flautas

Prep/Cook Time: 40 Min, Servings: 4, 0 WW Freestyle Smartpoint

Ingredients

- 1 Tbsp. butter
- 8 eggs, beaten
- ½ tsp. salt
- ¼ tsp. pepper
- 1 ½ tsp. cumin
- 1 tsp. chili powder
- 8 fajita size tortillas
- 4 oz cream cheese, softened
- 8 slices cooked bacon
- ½ cup shredded Mexican cheese
- ½ cup cotija cheese (or crumbled feta)

Avocado Crème

- 2 small avocados
- ½ cup sour cream
- 1 lime, juiced
- ½ tsp. salt
- ¼ tsp. pepper

Instructions

- In a large skillet, melt the butter over medium heat. Add the eggs and scramble until just cooked, about 3-4 minutes. Remove from heat and season with salt, pepper, cumin and chili powder.
- Spread cream cheese down the center of each tortilla. Lay one piece of bacon on top of cream cheese and top with scrambled eggs and shredded cheese.
- Tightly roll up tortillas.
- Place baking rack in the bowl in the low position and place 4 tortillas, seam side down on top.
- Tap the bake button and set temperature to 400°F and fry for 10-12 minutes, until tortillas are crispy.
- Remove and repeat with remaining tortillas.
- Meanwhile, add all avocado crème ingredients to a blender and blend on low-medium speed until smooth.
- Spread avocado crème over flautas and top with cotija cheese.

Nutrition Info : Calories 150 Calories from Fat 50, Fat 1g, Sodium 300mg, Potassium 702mg, Carbohydrates 23g, Fiber 6g, Protein 4g

Easy Air Fryer Omelette

Prep/Cook Time: 8 minutes!, Servings: 4, 4 WW Freestyle Smartpoint

Ingredients

- 2 eggs
- 1/4 cup milk
- Pinch of salt

- Fresh meat and veggies, diced (I used red bell pepper, green onions, ham and mushrooms)
- 1 teaspoon McCormick Good Morning Breakfast Seasoning – Garden Herb
- 1/4 cup shredded cheese (I used cheddar and mozzarella)

Instructions

- In a small bowl, mix the eggs and milk until well combined.
- Add a pinch of salt to the egg mixture.
- Add your veggies to the egg mixture.
- Pour the egg mixture into a well-greased 6?x3? pan.
- Place the pan into the basket of the air fryer.
- Cook at 350° Fahrenheit for 8-10 minutes.
- Halfway through cooking sprinkle the breakfast seasoning onto the eggs and sprinkle the cheese over the top.
- Use a thin spatula to loosen the omelette from the sides of the pan and transfer to a plate.
- Garnish with extra green onions, optional

Nutrition Info : Calories 201 Calories from Fat 9, Fat 4g, Sodium 302mg, Potassium 702mg, 0Carbohydrates 21g, Fiber 4g, Protein 6

Air Fryer Egg Rolls

Egg Rolls that you get at the Asian restaurant are so much more fattening because they are deep fried in oil and these air fryer egg rolls are so much healthier!

Prep/Cook Time: Servings: 8, 2 WW Freestyle Smartpoint

Ingredients

- 1 tsp minced ginger
- 4 1/2 cup(s) packaged coleslaw mix (shredded cabbage and carrots)
- 3 medium cooked scallion(s)
- 3 Tbsp low sodium soy sauce
- 1 1/2 tsp sesame oil
- 1 pound(s) uncooked ground chicken breast (can sub ground pork, turkey, or turkey sausage)
- 1 16 oz package of Egg Roll Wrappers (I only used 8 of them)
- 1 egg

Instructions

- Brown the sausage/meat in a medium non stick skillet until cooked all the way through and then add the ginger.
- Add soy sauce and sesame oil.
- Add full bag of coleslaw, stir till coated with sauce.

- Add chopped scallions, mix thoroughly and cook on medium high heat until the cole slaw has reduced by half.
- Set the egg roll mixture aside.
- Lay egg roll wrap in front of you so that it looks like a diamond.
- Place 3 tablespoons of filling in center of egg roll wrapper.
- Brush each edge with egg wash.
- Fold bottom point up over filling and roll once.
- Fold in right and left points.
- Finish rolling.
- Set aside and repeat with remaining filling.
- Heat Air Fryer to (370ºF).
- Set your stuffed egg rolls on the bottom of the air fryer basket and fry for 7 minutes or until they are golden brown.

Nutrition Info : Calories: 181Sugar: 1.4Fat: 4.1Saturated Fat: 1.4Carbohydrates: 21Fiber: 1.6

WW AIRFRYER VEGETARIAN RECIPES

Cheese and Veggie Egg Cups

Prep/Cook Time: 30 minutes, Servings: 4, 2 WW Freestyle Smartpoint

Ingredients

- Non-stick cooking spray
- 4 large eggs
- 1 cup diced veggies of choice
- 1 cup shredded cheese
- 4 Tbs half and half
- 1 Tbs chopped cilantro
- Salt and Pepper

Instructions

- Grease 4 ramekins
- In a medium bowl, whisk eggs, vegetables, half the cheese, half and half, cilantro, and salt and pepper together.
- Divide between the ramekins
- Place ramekins in the air-fryer basket, set temperature to 300 degrees F for 12 minutes.
- Top the cups with remaining cheese.
- Set air-fryer to 400 degrees F, cook 2 minutes until cheese is melted and lightly browned.
- Serve immediately.

Nutrition Info : Calories: 195kcal, Carbohydrates: 7g, Protein: 13g, Fat: 12g, Saturated Fat: 6g, Cholesterol: 191mg, Sodium: 265mg, Potassium: 197mg

Air Fryer Brussel Sprouts

Prep/Cook Time: 15 mins, Servings: 4 people, 5 WW Freestyle Smartpoint

Ingredients

- 3 c halved brussel sprouts
- 1 T olive oil
- 1/4 t salt
- 1/4 t pepper

Instructions

- Toss brussel sprouts with olive and salt/pepper.
- Place into air fryer basket.
- Set air fryer for 400 degrees F and cook 8-12 minutes.
- ENJOY!

Nutrition Info : Calories: 31kcal, Fat: 3g, Sodium: 145mg

Air Fried Tofu Italian Style

Prep/Cook Time: 20 minutes, Servings 2, 2 WW Freestyle Smartpoint

Ingredients
- 8 ounces extra-firm tofu
- 1 tablespoon soy sauce or tamari
- 1 tablespoon aquafaba or broth (see notes)
- 1/2 teaspoon dried oregano
- 1/2 teaspoon dried basil
- 1/2 teaspoon granulated garlic
- 1/4 teaspoon granulated onion

- black pepper to taste

Instructions

- Drain the tofu and cut it into three slices lengthwise. Put down a double layer of tea towels or paper towels, place the tofu slices on top, and cover with more towels. Place your hands over the tofu slices and press down, gently increasing pressure, to press enough water out that the towels are noticeably wet. (You can also use a tofu press for this, of course.)
- Return the tofu to the cutting board and cut each piece into about 10 cubes (one cut down the length and then 5 across works well.) Place the tofu in a large ziplock bag or bowl.
- Mix the remaining ingredients well. Pour over the tofu and gently turn the bag or stir the tofu until all sides are coated. Let it marinate at least 10 minutes--the longer you marinate it, the more flavorful it will be.
- Preheat your air fryer at 390-400F for about 3 minutes. Place the tofu in a single layer in the basket (leaving any marinade behind) and immediately reduce the temperature to around 350F. Air fry for 6 minutes. Use a thin, flexible spatula to loosen the tofu and turn it. Return it to the air fryer and begin checking at 4 minutes to see if it is golden overall and slightly darker at the edges but not overcooked or it will be tough.
- Use any way you like--my preference is in wraps with plenty of veggies and balsamic vinaigrette--but it's also good in pasta.

Nutrition Info : Calories 87 Calories from Fat 40, Fat 4.4g, Saturated Fat 1g, Sodium 452mg, Potassium 221mg, Carbohydrates 3.4g, Fiber 1.3g, Protein 10g

Vegan Air Fryer Buffalo Cauliflower

Prep/Cook Time: 25 minutes, Servings: 6, 4 WW Freestyle Smartpoint

Ingredients

- 1 large head cauliflower
- 1 cup unbleached all-purpose flour *(see note, GF flour works as well)
- 1 teaspoon vegan chicken bouillon granules
- 1/4 teaspoon cayenne pepper
- 1/4 teaspoon chili powder
- 1/4 teaspoon paprika
- 1/4 teaspoon dried chipotle chile flakes
- 1 cup soy milk
- canola oil spray
- 2 tablespoons nondairy butter
- 1/2 cup Frank's RedHot Original Cayenne Pepper Sauce or your favorite
- 2 cloves garlic, minced

Instructions

- Cut the cauliflower into bite-size pieces. Rinse and drain the cauliflower pieces.
- Combine the flour, bouillon granules, cayenne, chili powder, paprika, and chipotle flakes in a large bowl. Slowly whisk in the milk until a thick batter is formed.
- Spray the air fryer basket with canola oil and preheat the air fryer to 390°F for 10 minutes.

- While the air fryer is preheating, toss the cauliflower in the batter. Transfer the battered cauliflower to the air fryer basket. Cook for 20 minutes on 390°F. Using tongs, turn the cauliflower pieces at 10 minutes (don't be alarmed if they stick).
- After turning the cauliflower, heat the butter, hot sauce, and garlic in a small saucepan over medium high heat. Bring the mixture to a boil, reduce the heat to simmer, and cover.
- Once the cauliflower is cooked, transfer it to a large bowl. Pour the sauce over the cauliflower and toss gently with tongs. Serve immediately.

Nutrition Info : Calories 100 Calories from Fat 40, Fat 5.4g, Saturated Fat 2g, Sodium 452mg, 6Potassium 213mg, Carbohydrates 4g, Fiber 1.3g, Protein 10g

Air Fryer Roasted Cauliflower

Prep/Cook Time: 25 m, 2 servings, 8 WW Freestyle Smartpoint

Ingredients

- 3 cloves garlic
- 1 tablespoon peanut oil
- 1/2 teaspoon salt
- 1/2 teaspoon smoked paprika
- 4 cups cauliflower florets

Instructions

- Preheat an air fryer to 400 degrees F (200 degrees C).
- Cut garlic in half and smash with the blade of a knife. Place in a bowl with oil, salt, and paprika. Add cauliflower and turn to coat.
- Place the coated cauliflower in the bowl of the air fryer and cook to desired crispiness, about 15 minutes, shaking every 5 minutes.

Nutrition Info : 118 calories; 7 g fat; 12.4 g carbohydrates; 4.3 g protein; 0 mg cholesterol; 642 mg sodium.

Air Fryer Chickpeas

Prep/Cook Time: 14 mins, Servings: 4, 0 WW Freestyle Smartpoint

Ingredients

- 14 oz (400g) tin of chickpeas rinsed, drained and dried
- 2 tsp olive oil
- ½ tsp smoked paprika
- ½ tsp ground cumin
- salt

Instructions

- Pre heat air fryer to 390F / 200C.
- Mix all the ingredients together in a bowl.
- Add the chickpeas in to the air fryer basket.
- Cook for 12-15 mins turning half way through.

Tips for Making Crispy Air Fryer Chickpeas

- o For the chickpeas to crisp up, you have to make sure they are completely dry before you add the spiced oil mixture.
- o You can add an extra min or two for crispier chickpeas. Do keep an eye on them though as they burn very quickly.
- o You can easily vary the spices you add to the chickpeas to your taste.
- o These also work well with a dash of sriracha or chipotle sauce mixed in.
- o If you want to prep ahead the chickpeas, then do and let them cool down completely before keeping in an airtight container for a couple of hours.

Nutrition Info : Calories: 108kcal, Carbohydrates: 13g, Protein: 4g, Fat: 4g, Sodium: 276mg

Air Fryer Buffalo Cauliflower

Prep/Cook Time: 20 mins, Servings: 4, 3 WW Freestyle Smartpoint

Ingredients

For the Cauliflower

- 4 cups cauliflower florets – Each one should be approx. the size of two baby carrots, if you put the baby carrots side-by-side.
- 1 cup panko breadcrumbs mixed with 1 teaspoon sea salt – I would not use regular salt here. Sea salt grains are bigger, and they add a little extra crunch to the breading.

For the Buffalo Coating

- 1/4 cup melted vegan butter – 1/4 cup after melting
- 1/4 cup vegan Buffalo sauce – Check the ingredients for butter.

For Dipping

- vegan mayo – Cashew Ranch, or your favorite creamy salad dressing

Instructions

- o Melt the vegan butter in a mug in the microwave, then whisk in the buffalo sauce.
- o Holding by the stem, dip each floret in the butter/buffalo mixture, getting most of the floret coated in sauce. It's fine if a bit of the stem doesn't get saucy. Hold the floret over the mug until it pretty much stops dripping. A few drips are OK, but if it's raining sauce, your panko is going to get clumpy and stop sticking as well.
- o Dredge the dipped floret in the panko/salt mixture, coating as much as you like, then place in the air fryer. No need to worry about a single layer. Just drop it in there.
- o Air fry at 350F (do not preheat) for 14-17 minutes, shaking a few times, and checking their progress when you shake. Your cauliflower is done when the florets are a little bit browned.
- o Serve with your dipping sauce of choice.

Nutrition Info : Calories: 201kcal, Protein: 7g, Fat: 4g, Sodium: 303mg

Get Crispy Veggie Quesadillas in an Air Fryer

Prep/Cook Time: 40 Mins, Servings: 4, 7 WW Freestyle Smartpoint

Ingredients

- 4 (6-in.) sprouted whole-grain flour tortillas
- 4 ounces reduced-fat sharp Cheddar cheese, shredded (about 1 cup)
- 1 cup sliced red bell pepper
- 1 cup sliced zucchini
- 1 cup no-salt-added canned black beans, drained and rinsed Cooking spray
- 2 ounces plain 2% reduced-fat Greek yogurt
- 1 teaspoon lime zest plus 1 Tbsp. fresh juice (from 1 lime)
- 1/4 teaspoon ground cumin
- 2 tablespoons chopped fresh cilantro
- 1/2 cup drained refrigerated pico de gallo

Instructions

- Place tortillas on a work surface. Sprinkle 2 tablespoons shredded cheese over half of each tortilla. Top cheese on each tortilla with 1/4 cup each red pepper slices, zucchini slices, and black beans. Sprinkle evenly with remaining 1/2 cup cheese. Fold tortillas over to form half-moon shaped quesadillas. Lightly coat quesadillas with cooking spray, and secure with toothpicks.

- Lightly spray air fryer basket with cooking spray. Carefully place 2 quesadillas in the basket, and cook at 400°F until tortillas are golden brown and slightly crispy, cheese is melted, and vegetables are slightly softened, 10 minutes, turning quesadillas over halfway through cooking. Repeat with remaining quesadillas.
- While quesadillas cook, stir together yogurt, lime zest, lime juice, and cumin in a small bowl. To serve, cut each quesadilla into wedges and sprinkle with cilantro. Serve each with 1 tablespoon cumin cream and 2 tablespoons pico de gallo.

Nutrition Info : Calories 291 Fat 8g Satfat 4g Unsatfat 3g Protein 17g Carbohydrate 36g Fiber 8g Sugars 3g Added sugars 0g Sodium 518mg

Air-Fryer Vegan French "Toast"

Prep/Cook Time: 25 mins, Servings: 2, 7 WW Freestyle Smartpoint

Ingredients

- 1 block extra firm tofu
- 1/2 cup coconut flour
- 1/4 cup granulated Lakanto Monk Fruit Sweetener* (use coupon code ANNIE for 20% off)
- 1 Tbsp cinnamon

Instructions

- Drain tofu: remove tofu from package, and wrap the block of tofu in paper towels. Gently squeeze out

excess moisture, and set aside for about 10 minutes to allow it to continue draining.
- Combine coconut flour, granulated sweetener, and cinnamon in medium mixing bowl and mix.
- Slice tofu in half to create two square slabs that are about 1/2 inch thick. Slice each square in half diagonally.
- Preheat air fryer to 350F.
- Coat each piece of tofu in coconut flour mixture, and place in air fryer.
- Cook tofu for 7 minutes. Flip, and cook the other side for 7 more minutes.

Nutrition Info : Calories 258 Calories from Fat 117, Fat 13g, Saturated Fat 4g, Sodium 53mg, Potassium 634mg, Carbohydrates 15g, Fiber 10g, Sugar 3g, Protein 25g

Air Fryer Brussel Sprouts (Extra Crispy!)

Prep/Cook Time: 25 mins, Servings : 4, 5 WW Freestyle Smartpoint

Ingredients

- 1 pound fresh Brussels sprouts, washed, trimmed, and halved (large sprouts should be quartered)
- 2 teaspoons olive oil

Instructions

- Place the halved Brussels sprouts in a medium-size mixing bowl and add the oil. Toss to combine.
- Pour the sprouts into the base of your air fryer and set the temperature to 330°F.
- Bake for 18 minutes, stopping halfway through the baking process to open the drawer and shake the sprouts around.

o Serve the cooked sprouts hot.

Nutrition Info : Calories Per Serving: 69, Total Fat 2.7g, Saturated Fat 0.4g, Cholesterol 0mg, Sodium 28.3mg, Total Carbohydrate 10.1g, Dietary Fiber 4.3g, Sugars 2.5g, Protein 3.8g

Air Fryer Vegetable Kebabs

Prep/Cook Time:20 mins, Servings: 3, 0 WW Freestyle Smartpoint

Ingredients

- 2 bell peppers
- 1 eggplant
- 1 zuchini
- 1/2 onion
- salt and pepper to taste
- 6-inch skewers

Instructions

  o If using wooden skewers, place them in water for 10 minutes before using.
  o Cut all the veggies in about 1 inch pieces. Thread them on skewers and sprinkle with some salt and pepper
  o Preheat air fryer to 390F, add skewers and cook for 10 minutes.

Nutrition Info : Calories: 81kcal, Carbohydrates: 17g, Protein: 3g, Sodium: 12mg, Potassium: 714mg, Fiber: 7g, Sugar: 3g, Vitamin A: 2650IU, Vitamin C: 117.7mg, Calcium: 34mg, Iron: 0.9mg

Air Fryer Broccoli Parmesan

/Cook Time: 15 minutes, Servings: 4, 0 WW Freestyle Smartpoint

Ingredients

- 1 small head of broccoli, chopped into florets
- 2 garlic cloves, minced
- 2 Tbsp extra virgin olive oil
- 1/4 cup grated fresh parmesan cheese (more for topping, if desired)
- Optional : chili flakes for garnish

Instructions

- Pre heat your air fryer to 180C / 360F.
- In a bowl, mix the garlic, olive oil and parmesan cheese.
- Add the broccoli to the bowl.
- Use a spatula to mix it in, ensuring each floret is coated with the mixture. You want to make sure every bit of garlic and cheese is pressed into the nooks and crannies of the broccoli florets. This will help avoid it from falling off in the air fryer.
- Place the broccoli florets in the basket. If you like, you could sprinkle some extra cheese on top now. (I didn't in the broccoli photographed)
- Air fry for 3 to 5 minutes, until they are the desired crispiness.
- Sprinkle chili flakes on top for garnish, if desired.

Nutrition Info : Calories: 122 Total Fat: 8.8g Saturated Fat: 1.9g Trans Fat: 0g Cholesterol: 3.6mg Sodium: 122mg Carbohydrates: 8.2g Fiber: 3g Sugar: 2g Protein: 5.2g

Blackened Air Fryer Salmon with Cucumber-Avocado Salsa

Prep/Cook Time: 29 minutes, Servings: 4 Servings, 3 Weight Watchers SP

Ingredients

The salmon:

- 1 tablespoon sweet paprika
- 1/2 teaspoon cayenne pepper
- 1 teaspoon garlic powder
- 1 teaspoon dried oregano
- 1 teaspoon dried thyme
- 3/4 teaspoon kosher salt
- 1/8 teaspoon freshly ground black pepper
- Olive oil spray
- 4 (6 oz each) wild salmon fillets

The salsa:

- 2 tablespoons chopped red onion
- 1 1/2 tablespoons fresh lemon juice
- 1 teaspoon extra virgin olive oil
- 1/4 + 1/8 teaspoon kosher salt
- Freshly ground black pepper
- 4 Persian (mini) cucumbers* diced
- 6 ounces Hass avocado (1 large) diced

Instructions

The salmon:

- o In a small bowl, combine the paprika, cayenne, garlic powder, oregano, thyme, salt and black pepper.
- o Spray both sides fo the fish with oil and rub all over. Coat the fish all over with the spices.
- o Preheat the air fryer to 400 degrees F.
- o Working in batches, arrange the salmon fillets skin side down in the air fryer basket.
- o Cook until the fish flakes easily with a fork, 5 to 7 minutes, depending on the thickness of the fish. (For a toaster oven-style air fryer, the temperature and timing remain the same.)
- o Serve topped with the salsa.

The salsa: In a medium bowl, combine the red onion, lemon juice, olive oil, salt and pepper to taste. Let stand for 5 minutes, then add the cucumbers and avocado.

Nutrition Info : Calories: 340kcal, Carbohydrates: 8g, Protein: 35g, Fat: 18.5g, Saturated Fat: 3g, Cholesterol: 94mg, Sodium: 396mg, Fiber: 4g, Sugar: 2g

Vegan Air Fryer Buffalo Cauliflower

Prep/Cook Time: 25 minutes, Servings: 4, 5 Weight Watchers SP

Ingredients

- 1 large head cauliflower
- 1 cup unbleached all-purpose flour *(see note, GF flour works as well)
- 1 teaspoon vegan chicken bouillon granules
- 1/4 teaspoon cayenne pepper
- 1/4 teaspoon chili powder
- 1/4 teaspoon paprika
- 1/4 teaspoon dried chipotle chile flakes
- 1 cup soy milk
- canola oil spray
- 2 tablespoons nondairy butter
- 1/2 cup Frank's RedHot Original Cayenne Pepper Sauce or your favorite
- 2 cloves garlic, minced

Instructions

- Cut the cauliflower into bite-size pieces. Rinse and drain the cauliflower pieces.
- Combine the flour, bouillon granules, cayenne, chili powder, paprika, and chipotle flakes in a large bowl. Slowly whisk in the milk until a thick batter is formed.
- Spray the air fryer basket with canola oil and preheat the air fryer to 390°F for 10 minutes.
- While the air fryer is preheating, toss the cauliflower in the batter. Transfer the battered cauliflower to the air fryer basket. Cook for 20 minutes on 390°F. Using

- tongs, turn the cauliflower pieces at 10 minutes (don't be alarmed if they stick).
- After turning the cauliflower, heat the butter, hot sauce, and garlic in a small saucepan over medium high heat. Bring the mixture to a boil, reduce the heat to simmer, and cover.
- Once the cauliflower is cooked, transfer it to a large bowl. Pour the sauce over the cauliflower and toss gently with tongs. Serve immediately.

Nutrition Info : Calories: 191 Total Fat: 13g Saturated Fat: 4g Trans Fat: 0g Unsaturated Fat: 6g Cholesterol: 0mg Sodium: 230mg Carbohydrates: 2g Fiber: 8g Sugar: 8g Protein: 13g

Air-Fried Vegan Tofu

Prep/Cook Time: 30 minutes, Servings: 4, 4 WW Freestyle Smartpoint

Ingredients

- 15 ounces extra-firm tofu
- 2 teaspoons olive oil
- 1/4 teaspoon salt

Instructions

- Remove tofu from it's container. Wrap in paper towels or a kitchen towel and stand over the sink and gently press tofu to remove excess liquid. Cut into 1/2? cubes. Use a paper towel to dry the cubes. Drizzle with olive oil and toss gently to coat each piece.
- Preheat air fryer to 375F and set the timer for 18 minutes. Allow the air fryer to heat up. Remove the basket and spray with vegetable cooking spray. Add

- the tofu cubes and spray the top with vegetable cooking spray.
    o Every 5 minutes, remove the basket and stir the tofu by shaking the basket so that each piece is browned equally. Cook for 15 – 18 minutes, or until desired crispiness is reached.
    o Serve fried tofu over rice with steamed veggies. Drizzle with any extra marinade. Or serve fried tofu as an appetizer by serving with a dipping sauce.
    o Transfer any unused tofu to a sealed container and refrigerate for up to 7 days.

Nutrition Info : Calories 78, Total Fat 0, Saturated Fat 0, Trans Fat, Cholesterol 0

WW AIRFRYER FISH & SEAFOOD RECIPES

Weight Watcher Oven Fried Fish

Prep/Cook Time: 20mins, Serves: 6, 3 Ww Freestyle Smartpoint

Ingredients

- 1 1/2 lbs tilapia fillets or 1 1/2 lbs other white fish
- 1/4 cup white cornmeal (or yellow)
- 1/4 cup dry breadcrumbs (I use seasoned)
- 1/2 teaspoon dried dill
- 1/2 teaspoon salt
- 1/8 teaspoon pepper
- 1/2 teaspoon paprika
- 1/3 cup skim milk
- 3 tablespoons butter, melted

Instructions

- Preheat oven to 450 degrees.
- In a shallow dish, like a pie plate, combine all dry ingredients.
- Place milk in another shallow dish.
- Dip fish in milk, then in crumb mixture.
- Place in pan coated with cooking spray.
- Drizzle with melted butter.
- Bake for 10 minute or until fish flakes apart with fork.

Nutrition Info : Calories: 356kcal, Carbohydrates: 8g, Protein: 33g, Fat: 13g, Cholesterol: 121mg, Sodium: 373mg, Sugar: 1g

Healthy Baked Fish Sticks with Lemon Caper Sauce

Prep/Cook Time: 30 mins, 4 servings, 4 WW Freestyle Smartpoint

Ingredients

Lemon Caper Sauce:

- 1/4 cup fat free plain Greek yogurt
- 3 tablespoons light mayonnaise
- 1 tablespoon drained capers
- 1 tablespoon fresh minced chives
- 1 teaspoon fresh lemon juice
- 1/4 teaspoon kosher salt
- 1/8 teaspoon black pepper

For the Fish Sticks:

- cooking spray, I use a mister
- 1 pound Alaskan skinless cod fillet, about 1-inch thick (thawed if frozen)
- 3 large egg whites
- 1 tablespoon Dijon mustard
- 1/2 lemon, squeezed
- 1/8 teaspoon paprika
- 1/4 teaspoon kosher salt
- 1/8 teaspoon black pepper

For the crumbs:

- 1 cup plain or gluten-free Panko crumbs
- 1 1/2 teaspoons Old Bay seasoning
- 2 teaspoons dried parsley flakes
- 1/2 teaspoon paprika

Instructions

o Preheat the air fryer to 370F.

- In batches, transfer to the air fryer basket in a single layer and cook until the crumbs are golden and the fish is cooked through, 7 to 8 minutes, turning halfway.

Nutrition Info: Calories: 229kcal, Carbohydrates: 15g, Protein: 31g, Fat: 4g, Saturated Fat: 0.5g, Cholesterol: 63mg, Sodium: 709mg, Fiber: 1g, Sugar: 2g

Air Fryer Tuna Cakes Recipe

Prep/Cook Time: 15 mins, Serves: 1, 3 WW Freestyle Smartpoint

Ingredients

- 1 3oz. can tuna in water
- 1 tablespoon flour
- 1 teaspoon light mayonnaise
- 1/8 teaspoon garlic powder
- 1/8 teaspoon dried dill
- 1/8 teaspoon salt
- 1/8 teaspoon black pepper

Instructions

- Drain water from tuna
- In a small bowl, mix all ingredients together until well blended. Will be slightly moist, but should be able to form patties.
- Divide into 4 equal portions, and create small circular patties.
- Lay in the basket of air fryer in a single layer.
- Following your air fryer Instructions, close and set to 380 degrees for 10 minutes. You may flip each patty

halfway through if preferred, but it will cook well either way.

Nutrition Info : Calories: 300kcal, Carbohydrates: 15g, Protein: 31g, Fat: 4g, Saturated Fat:0.5g, Cholesterol: 63mg, Sodium: 709mg, Fiber: 1g, Sugar: 2g

Air-Fried Crumbed Fish

Prep/Cook Time 22 m, 4 servings, 5 WW Freestyle Smartpoint

Ingredients

- 1 cup dry bread crumbs
- 1/4 cup vegetable oil
- 4 flounder fillets
- 1 egg, beaten
- 1 lemon, sliced

Instructions

o Preheat an air fryer to 350 degrees F (180 degrees C).
o Mix bread crumbs and oil together in a bowl. Stir until mixture becomes loose and crumbly.
o Dip fish fillets into the egg; shake off any excess. Dip fillets into the bread crumb mixture; coat evenly and fully.
o Lay coated fillets gently in the preheated air fryer. Cook until fish flakes easily with a fork, about 12 minutes. Garnish with lemon slices.

Nutrition Info : 354 calories; 17.7 g fat; 22.5 g carbohydrates; 26.9 g protein; 107 mg cholesterol; 309 mg sodium.

PointsPlus "Fried" Catfish with Potato Sticks Recipe

Prep/Cook Time: 45 mins, Servings: 4, 3 WW Freestyle Smartpoint

Ingredients

- Nonstick cooking spray
- 1 ¼ pounds red potatoes, scrubbed
- ½ teaspoon salt
- ½ teaspoon black pepper
- 1 large egg
- ¼ cup yellow cornmeal
- 2 tablespoons finely chopped fresh parsley
- Four 5-ounce catfish fillets
- 4 lemon wedges

Instructions

- Preheat oven to 400 degrees. Spray 2 baking sheets with nonstick spray.
- Cut potatoes into ½-by-2-inch sticks; rinse under cold running water and pat dry with paper towels. Spread in single layer on one of prepared baking sheets; spray with nonstick spray. Bake until potatoes are golden brown and crispy, about 30 minutes. Immediately sprinkle with ¼ teaspoon of salt and ¼ teaspoon of pepper.
- Meanwhile, lightly beat egg in pie plate. Mix together cornmeal, parsley, remaining ¼ teaspoon salt and remaining ¼ teaspoon pepper on sheet of wax paper. Dip catfish, one fillet at a time, in egg, then coat with cornmeal mixture, pressing so it adheres.
- Place fish on remaining prepared baking sheet; lightly spray with nonstick spray. Bake until golden brown and just opaque in center, about 12 minutes. Serve with potato sticks and lemon wedges.

Nutrition Info : 325 calories; 16.7 g fat; 22.5 g carbohydrates; 26.9 g protein; 107 mg cholesterol; 309 mg sodium.

Soy-Glazed Fish with Stir-Fried Spinach

Prep/Cook Time: 20 min, Servings: 4, 1 WW Freestyle Smartpoint

Ingredients

- garlic clove(s)
- 2 medium clove(s), minced uncooked scallion(s)
- 2 Tbsp, minced cilantro
- 2 Tbsp, fresh, minced low sodium soy sauce
- 2 Tbsp ginger root
- 1 Tbsp, fresh, finely minced cooking spray
- 5 spray(s), divided toasted sesame oil
- 1 Tbsp, divided uncooked Pacific cod
- 1 pound(s), or other cod, washed and dried fresh spinach
- 1 pound(s), baby leaves

Instructions

- In a small bowl, combine garlic, scallions, cilantro, soy sauce and ginger; set aside.
- Coat a medium skillet with cooking spray; add 1 1/2 teaspoons oil and heat over medium-high heat. Add fish; cook until moisture starts to appear on top of fish, about 3 to 5 minutes (depending on thickness of fish).
- Carefully flip fish; pour garlic-soy mixture over top. Cook until fish is no longer translucent in middle, about 3 minutes more. (If sauce starts to stick to bottom of pan, add a little broth or water.)
- Meanwhile, coat a large skillet with cooking spray; add remaining 1 1/2 teaspoons oil and heat over medium-high heat. Add spinach; cook, tossing spinach

constantly, until spinach is wilted, about 3 to 4 minutes. Spoon spinach on a serving plate and place fish on top. Servings s about 3 1/2 ounces fish and 3/4 cup spinach per serving.

Nutrition Info : 300 calories; 16.7 g fat; 20.5 g carbohydrates; 30.9 g protein; 107 mg cholesterol

Air Fryer Fish and Chips Healthy

Prep/Cook Time: Servings : 2, 2 WW Freestyle Smartpoint

Ingredients

- 2 4-6 oz Tilapia Filets
- 2 tablespoons of flour
- 1 egg
- 1/2 cup of panko bread crumbs
- Old Bay Seasoning
- salt and pepper
- Frozen Crinkle Cut Fries such as Ore Ida

Instructions

- Gather 3 small bowls. In one bowl add the flour, in the 2nd bowl add the egg and beat it with a wire whisk, in the 3rd bowl add the panko bread crumbs and Old Bay Seasoning.
- Take the fish and dredge it in the flour, then the egg, and next in the bread crumbs. Add to the air fryer a long with 15 frozen french fries. Air Fry for 15 minutes at 390 degrees.

Nutrition Info : Calories: 219, Sugar: 1, Sodium: 356, Fat: 5, Saturated Fat: 3, Carbohydrates: 18, Fiber: 1, Protein: 25

Extra Crispy Air Fryer Bacon Recipe

Prep/Cook Time: Servings: 8, 3 WW Freestyle Smartpoint

Ingredients

- 1 Pound Bacon Thick Cut

Instructions

- Preheat air fryer at 400 degrees.
- Spray air fryer basket with nonstick cooking spray. Place the bacon in the air fryer basket in a single layer.
- Cook bacon for 8 to 10 minutes, flipping halfway. Remove bacon and place on paper towels. Keep warm.
- Repeat until all bacon is cooked.

Nutrition Info : Calories: 236kcal, Carbohydrates: 1g, Protein: 7g, Fat: 23g, Saturated Fat: 8g, Cholesterol: 37mg, Sodium: 375mg, Potassium: 112mg, Vitamin A: 21IU, Calcium: 3mg, Iron: 1mg

Air Fryer Fish

Easy air fryer fish that is crispy and golden from the outside, soft and moist from the inside. Cooked in just 15 minutes!

Prep/Cook Time: 20 minutes, Servings: 4,

Ingredients

- 8 (800 grams) fish fillets
- 1 tbsp olive oil
- 1 cup 50 grams bread crumbs If following Gluten free diet, use gluten free breadcrumbs.
- 1/2 tsp paprika
- 1/4 tsp dried chili powder
- 1/4 tsp ground black pepper
- 1/4 tsp garlic powder
- 1/4 tsp onion powder
- 1/2 tsp salt

Instructions

- If using frozen fish fillets, defrost them. Drizzle with olive oil, and mix the fish to make sure that it's well coated with oil.
- In a shallow dish, mix the bread crumbs with paprika, chili powder, black pepper, garlic powder, onion powder and salt.
- Coat each fish fillet in bread crumbs, and transfer to your air fryer basket.
- Cook in the air fryer at 390F or 200C for 12-15 minutes. After the first 8-10 minutes, open the air fryer and flip the fish fillets on the other side then continue cooking.

Nutrition Info : Calories: 153kcal, Carbohydrates: 11g, Protein: 21g, Fat: 3g, Cholesterol: 50mg, Sodium: 269mg, Potassium: 302mg, Fiber: 1g

Air Fryer garlic lime shrimp kabobs

Prep/Cook Time:13 mins, Servings: 2, Zero WW Freestyle Smartpoint

Ingredients

- 1 cup raw shrimp
- 1 garlic clove
- 1 lime
- 1/8 teaspoon salt
- freshly ground pepper
- 5 6 inch wooden skewers

Instructions

- Soak wooden skewers in water for 20 minutes.
- Thaw shrimp if frozen. Preheat the Air fryer to 350F.
- Mix shrimp with juiced lime and minced garlic. Add salt and pepper.
- Put shrimp on each skewer(i was able to put 5 on each). Place in the air fryer for 8 minutes, flip half way through.
- Serve with chopped cilantro on top and your favorite dip.

Nutrition Info : Calories 76, Cholesterol 161mg, Sodium 643mg, Potassium 85mg, Carbohydrates 4g, Protein 13g

Air Fryer Parmesan Shrimp

Prep/Cook Time: 10 minutes, Servings: 5, 2 WW Freestyle Smartpoint

Ingredients

- 2 pounds jumbo cooked shrimp, peeled and deveined
- 4 cloves garlic, minced
- 2/3 cup parmesan cheese, grated
- 1 teaspoon pepper
- 1/2 teaspoon oregano
- 1 teaspoon basil
- 1 teaspoon onion powder
- 2 tablespoons olive oil
- Lemon, quartered

Instructions

- In a large bowl, combine garlic, parmesan cheese, pepper, oregano, basil, onion powder and olive oil.
- Gently toss shrimp in mixture until evenly-coated.
- Spray air fryer basket with non-stick spray and place shrimp in basket.
- Cook at 350 degrees for 8-10 minutes or until seasoning on shrimp is browned.
- Squeeze the lemon over the shrimp before serving.

Notes : If using an oven, bake at 400 degrees for 6-8 minutes.

Nutrition Info : Calories: 100kcal, Carbohydrates: 5g, Protein: 16g, Cholesterol: 150mg | Sodium: 222mg, Potassium: 65mg

Air Fryer Weight Watchers Crab Wontons

Prep/Cook Time: 30 minutes, Servings: 48 wontons, 1 WW Smart Point

Ingredients

- 1 cup crab meat or imitation crab meat
- 8 oz fat-free cream cheese
- 2 tsp Worcestershire sauce
- 1/2 teaspoon light soy sauce
- 1 tbsp minced garlic
- 48 Wonton Wrappers

Instructions

- Mix the cream cheese, crab, Worcestershire sauce, soy sauce, and garlic together in a bowl.
- Spoon 1 teaspoon of cream cheese mixture in the middle of each wonton wrapper.
- Wipe the edges of the wonton wrappers with water.
- Bring all 4 corners together in the center and seal.
- Spray the bottom of the fryer basket with cooking spray.
- Put as many as your air fryer can hold without over crowding.
- Spray the tops of the wontons with cooking spray.
- Cook in the Air Fryer at 390 degrees 7-10 minutes (Flipping over halfway through.)
- Serve warm!

Nutrition Info : Calories: 150kcal, Carbohydrates: 7g, Protein: 14g, Cholesterol: 114mg | Sodium: 232mg, Potassium: 65mg

Easy Baked Tilapia

Prep/Cook Time: 20 mins, Servings: 4, 2 WW Freestyle Smart Points

Ingredients

- ½ cup Italian style Panko breadcrumbs
- ¼ cup Parmesan cheese
- 1 pound tilapia fillets

Instructions

- Preheat oven to 425°F.
- In a shallow bowl, combine breadcrumbs and Parmesan cheese.
- Rinse off the tilapia fillets. Coat damp tilapia fillets with the crumb mixture.
- Place the coated fillets on a cooking sheet, or stone.
- Spray the fillets with cooking spray. (optional step)
- Bake for 10-12 minutes

Nutrition Info : Calories: 80kcal, Protein: 12g, Cholesterol: 100mg, Sodium: 342mg, Potassium: 40mg

Cilantro Lime Air Fryer Shrimp Skewers

Prep/Cook Time:13 mins, Servings: 4, zero Freestyle Points

Ingredients

- 1/2 lb (225g) raw shrimp peeled and deveined
- 1/2 tsp garlic purée
- 1/2 tsp paprika
- 1/2 tsp ground cumin
- Juice of 1 lemon
- Salt to taste
- 1 tbsp of chopped cilantro (fresh coriander leaves)

Instructions

Air Fryer Instructions:

- Soak 6 wooden skewers for 15-20 mins before needed.
- Preheat air fryer to 350 F (180C).
- Mix lemon Juice, garlic, paprika, cumin and salt in a bowl. Add shrimp and stir to evenly coat.
- Thread shrimp onto the skewers.
- Place skewers in air fryer and make sure they are not touching.
- Cook for 5-8 mins, turning skewers halfway through the cook time. Since air fryer temperatures can vary, start with less time and then add more as needed.
- Transfer shrimp to a plate and serve with chopped cilantro (coriander) and extra lime slices.

Grill Instructions:

- Preheat the grill (or barbeque) to medium.
- Oil the grill plate (make sure use an oil approved for your dietary considerations).
- Place shrimp on a griddle on the hot barbeque or grill.
- Cook for 2-3 mins on each side until they are cooked through.
- Transfer to a plate and serve.

Nutrition Info : Calories: 59kcal, Protein: 11g, Cholesterol: 142mg, Sodium: 441mg, Potassium: 45mg

Air Fryer Bang Bang Shrimp (with lightened up sauce)

Prep/Cook Time: 23 mins, Servings: 6, 6 WW Freestyle Points

Ingredients

- pound large cooked shrimp peeled, deveined, and tails removed, defrosted
- olive oil spray

For the coating:

- 1/4 cup flour
- 1 tsp salt
- 1/2 tsp pepper
- 1/2 tsp paprika
- 1/4 tsp garlic powder
- 1 cup panko
- 1/2 cup cornstarch
- 2 medium eggs
- 1 TBS water

For the Bang Bang Sauce:

- 1/3 cup Greek yogurt, (plain, 2% or nonfat)
- 2 TBS light mayonnaise
- 2 TBS sriracha
- 2 TBS sugar
- 1 TBS rice vinegar

For Garnish: chopped green onions or chopped cilantro, optional

Instructions

To coat the shrimp:

- Setup all of the ingredients; it's easiest to make the air fryer bang bang shrimp in somewhat of an assembly line.
- Place flour into a large Ziploc bag. Place eggs and water into a small bowl and beat together. Place cornstarch, panko breadcrumbs, salt, pepper, garlic powder, and paprika in a shallow container and mix well.
- Add the shrimp to the plastic bag with the flour and toss to coat. Tap off any excess flour off before the next step.
- Add a few shrimp to the egg wash, and toss to coat completely.
- Add the shrimp to the breadcrumb mixture, toss and press the coating into the shrimp, being sure it sticks. Repeat for all of the shrimp.
- Wash hands with Lava® Soap to remove all of the grime from your hands!

To cook the Air Fryer Bang Bang Shrimp:

- o Place the shrimp into the air fryer, adding only as many as will fit in a single layer. Give a quick spray of olive oil over the tops of the shrimp, then close the air fryer.
- o Set the temperature at 400 degrees and the timer to 5 minutes. When the time is up, carefully flip the shrimp over, spray with olive oil, then close and set again to 400 degrees and set the timer for 3 minutes.
- o Remove when the time is up, then repeat until the rest of the shrimp are cooked.

For the sauce: In a small bowl, add Greek yogurt, mayonnaise, sugar, sriracha, and rice vinegar. Whisk to combine; place in fridge until ready to serve.

To serve: Place cooked bang bang shrimp on a tray, then top with bang bang sauce right before serving. Add chopped green onion or chopped cilantro over the top of the bang bang shrimp and enjoy!

Nutrition Info : 226 calories, 4 grams of fat, 27 grams carbohydrates, 20 grams protein, 1 gram fiber, 6 grams sugar.

Low Fat Parmesan Crusted Tilapia

Prep/Cook Time: 20 mins, Servings:4, 3 Weight Watchers Points

Ingredients

- 4 whole Tilapia Filets 2-3 ounces each

- ¼ Cup Panko Bread Crumbs I use gluten free
- 1 Tablespoon Grated Parmesan
- 1/8 Teaspoon Garlic Powder
- 1/8 Teaspoon Onion Powder
- 1/8 Teaspoon Cayenne Pepper
- 1/8 Teaspoon Dill Weed

Instructions

- Spray a baking dish with non-stick cooking spray
- Preheat oven to 375 degrees
- In shallow dish together bread crumbs, Parmesan and seasonings
- Rinse and pat dry tilapia fillets.
- Press tilapia gently into bread crumb mixture lightly coating both sides.
- Place into baking dish
- Bake at 375 degrees for 15 minutes
- Place oven on broil and cook for additional 2-3 minutes or until tops are golden brown (watch closely as this can burn very quickly).
- Makes 4 servings of 3 Weight Watchers Points Each.

Nutrition Info : 190 calories, 5 grams of fat, 25 grams carbohydrates, 22 grams protein

Oven Fried Shrimp Recipe (5 WW points)

Prep/Cook Time: 45 mins, Servings: 4, 3 W W Freestyle SmartPoints

Ingredients

- 16 oz of fresh or frozen shrimp
- 2 tablespoons of grated Parmesan cheese
- 3/4 cup of Panko breadcrumbs
- 1 large egg

- 1 egg white
- 1 1/2 teaspoons of Cajun seasoning
- 1/2 teaspoon of salt
- 1/4 teaspoon of black pepper
- cooking spray

Instructions

- We like to use fresh shrimp when ever possible. So if you go with fresh shrimp with the shell still on it, you'll need to peel it first. Remove the entire shell.
- If you use frozen shrimp, thaw it first by running the shrimp under cool water until completely thawed.
- Preheat oven to 400 and spray a baking sheet with cooking spray.
- In a bowl, mix Panko breadcrumbs, salt, pepper, Parmesan cheese and Cajun seasoning.
- In a separate bowl, whisk together the 1 egg and the 1 egg white.
- Dip each shrimp in the egg first and then coat in the breadcrumb mixture.
- Place shrimp on greased baking sheet and bake for about 15 minutes (for large shrimp).

Nutrition Info : Calories: 195kcal, Carbohydrates: 7g, Protein: 13g, Fat: 12g, Saturated Fat: 6g

Air Fryer Shrimp Egg Rolls

Prep/Cook Time: 30 mins, Servings: 5, 5 WW FreeStyle SP

Ingredients

- 1 teaspoon toasted sesame oil
- 1 teaspoon fresh ground ginger
- 3 garlic cloves, minced
- 1 cup chopped carrots
- 1/2 cup sliced green onion
- 2 tablespoons soy sauce
- 1/2 tablespoon sugar
- 1/4 cup chicken or vegetable broth
- 3 cups coleslaw mix or shredded cabbage
- 10 large cooked shrimp, cut into small pieces
- 10 egg roll wrappers
- 1 egg, beaten

Instructions

- Heat oil in a large skillet over medium heat. Add ginger and garlic and cook for 30 seconds.
- Add carrots and green onion to pan and sauté for 2 minutes.
- Meanwhile, whisk together soy sauce, sugar and broth.
- Mix in soy sauce mixture, coleslaw mix/cabbage, and shrimp to the pan of veges and cook 5 minutes.
- Remove pan from heat and allow to cool for about 15 minutes and strain the liquid in a strainer.

- As the coleslaw/vegetable mixture is cooling, preheat the air fryer to 390°F.
- Place the egg roll wrappers on a work surface. Top each with 3 tablespoons veggie/shrimp mixture.
- Brush some egg on the edges of the wrapper. Roll up the wrappers, folding over the sides so the filling is contained. Brush the egg on the outside of each egg roll right before you will be adding them to the air fryer. (If you brush it on and let it sit the egg roll gets soft and can rip).
- Spray the air fryer basket with cooking spray. Carefully add 3-4 egg rolls to the air fryer basket at a time. Brush tops of egg rolls with egg.
- Air fry 8-9 minutes, or until brown and crunchy on the outside.
- Serve immediately.

Nutrition Info : Calories 240 Calories from Fat 18, Fat 2g, Cholesterol 80mg, Sodium 913mg, Carbohydrates 39g, Fiber 2g, Sugar 4g, Protein 12g

Low Carb Meatballs in the Airfryer

Prep/Cook Time: 20 minutes, Servings: 4, 5 WW FreeStyle SP

Ingredients

- 1 pound ground chicken
- 1/4 cup chopped cilantro
- 1 teaspoon fresh mint
- 1 tablespoon lime juice
- 1 tablespoon curry paste
- 1 tablespoon fish sauce
- 2 garlic cloves, minced
- 2 teaspoons minced ginger
- 1/2 teaspoon salt
- 1/2 teaspoon black pepper
- 1/4 teaspoon red pepper flakes

Instructions

- In a large bowl, mix the ground chicken, culinary paste (or list of spices if preferred), and cilantro until combined
- Form the mixture into 16 meatballs and place in single layer in the air fryer basket.
- Set air fryer to 400°F and cook for 10 minutes, turning meatballs halfway through cooking time
- Use a meat thermometer to ensure internal cooking temp of 165°F

Notes : Cooking in one layer is key to to air fryer recipes so either cooking batches if necessary or invest in an air fryer rack that will allow you to cook in two layers at once.

Nutrition Info : Calories: 152kcal, Protein: 23.2g, Fat: 6g

Air Fryer Fish And Chips

Prep/Cook Time:45 mins, Servings: 4 servings

Ingredients
- 1 lb fish fillet (cod, tilapia, catfish)
- 1 cup breadcrumbs (i used panko)
- 1 egg
- 1/4 cup flour
- 1 tspn salt
- 2 tbspn oil
- 2 russet potatoes

Instructions
- Cut potatoes in wedges or like french fries. In a bowl, toss together potatoes. salt and oil.
- Add potatoes in to your air fryer basket and cook on 400F for 20 minutes, shaking twice. Once done remove from the basket.
- Meanwhile, prepare the fish. In a shallow bowl add flour, in a second bowl add beaten egg and in the third bowl add Panko. Working with one piece at a time, dredge fish fillet first in flour, then in egg, and then in breadcrumbs.
- Add fish to the air fryer and set it to 330F for 15 minutes. Check on it halfway through and flip if needed.
- Serve together immediately with any sauce(I used Spicy Aioli)

Nutrition Info : Calories 409 Calories from Fat 99, Fat 11g, Saturated Fat 1g, Cholesterol 97mg, Sodium 374mg, Potassium 854mg, Carbohydrates 44g, Fiber 2g, Protein 30g

WW AIRFRYER POULTRY RECIPES

Buffalo Style Air Fryer Chicken Wings

Prep/Cook Time: 1 hour 20 mins, Servings : 4, 4 Smart Points

Ingredients

- 1 lb. Chicken Wings (fresh or frozen)
- 1/2 cup Frank's Hot Sauce
- Fat Free Blue Cheese (optional)

Instructions

- Preheat air fryer for 3-5 minutes on 380°.
- Place chicken wings in a single layer in air fryer.
- Air fry for 12 minutes on 380°.
- Flip wings and air fry for another 12 minutes.
- You can add your sauce now, or at the end of your cooking.
- After the 12 minutes is done - turn the temperature up to 400° and cook for 5 more minutes
- Be sure the internal temperature of the wings are 165° before removing
- If you did not add your sauce during the cooking, then place in bowl and add your preferred sauce and shake or toss until wings are covered.

Nutrition Info : Calories 348 Calories from Fat 85, Fat 12g, Saturated Fat 1.3g, Cholesterol 97mg, Sodium 333mg, Potassium 782mg, Carbohydrates 47g, Fiber 1g, Protein 34g

Air Fryer Chicken Nuggets

Prep/Cook Time: 20 mins, 4 Servings, 3 Freestyle Points

Ingredients

- 16 oz 2 large skinless boneless chicken breasts, cut into even 1-inch bite sized pieces
- 1/2 teaspoon kosher salt and black pepper, to taste
- 2 teaspoons olive oil
- 6 tablespoons whole wheat Italian seasoned breadcrumbs
- 2 tablespoons panko
- 2 tablespoons grated parmesan cheese
- olive oil spray, I used my Misto

Instructions

- Preheat air fryer to 400°F for 8 minutes.
- Put the olive oil in one bowl and the breadcrumbs, panko and parmesan cheese in another.
- Season chicken with salt and pepper, then put in the bowl with the olive oil and mix well so the olive oil evenly coats all of the chicken.
- Put a few chunks of chicken at a time into the breadcrumb mixture to coat, then on the basket.
- Lightly spray the top with olive oil spray then air fry 8 minutes, turning halfway. Until golden.

Nutrition Info : Calories: 188kcal, Carbohydrates: 8g, Protein: 25g, Fat: 4.5g, Saturated Fat: 1g, Cholesterol: 57mg, Sodium: 427mg, Sugar: 0.5g

Air Fryer Whole Chicken

Prep/Cook Time: 55 minutes, Servings: 4,

Ingredients

- 3 lbs 1.3 kg whole chicken

For the marinade

- 1/4 cup 60 ml Olive oil
- 1 tbsp Ginger
- 1 clove Garlic
- 1 tbsp Thyme leaves
- 1 tbsp Smoked paprika
- 2 tsp Salt
- 1/4 tsp ground black pepper

To stuff the chicken
- 3 cloves garlic
- bunch thyme leaves
- 1 lemon sliced

Instructions

To make the marinade: Whisk the ingredients until well combined.

To cook the chicken:

- Prepare the chicken. Remove the chicken giblets, rinse the chicken inside out and remove any excess fat or pin feathers. Using kitchen towels, pat the chicken dry. Using kitchen string, tie the legs together.

- o Stuff the inside of the chicken with a bunch of thyme, lemon wedges, and garlic cloves.
- o Then using a brush, brush the marinade all over the chicken and make sure that the chicken is well coated.
- o Transfer to the air fryer. Cook 200c/390f for 30 minutes. Then flip the chicken over, and cook for an additional 10 minutes.

Notes
- Make sure that the chicken is completely covered with the marinade before cooking to get more flavor.
- If your chicken is smaller/bigger than the one in this recipe, the cooking time will be different.
- The air fryer that I've used to roast a whole chicken, is this 4.2L air fryer so the chicken fit perfectly. It's great for families and for cooking bigger amounts of food. If your chicken won't fit, you can cut it up into smaller pieces or just remove the backbone (save the backbone to make homemade stock later!).
- Start with the chicken breast side up, then after 30 minutes of cooking flip the chicken and cook for an additional 10 minutes.
- Make sure that you check the doneness of the chicken before removing it from the air fryer. You don't want to undercook or overcook the meat.
- Let the chicken rest for 5-10 minutes before serving.

Nutrition Info : Calories: 169kcal, Carbohydrates: 4g, Protein: 25g, Fat: 6g, Saturated Fat: 1g, Cholesterol: 118mg, Sodium: 901mg, Potassium: 372mg, Fiber: 1g, Sugar: 1g

Crispy Air Fryer Chicken Breast

Easy crispy and golden air fryer chicken breast chicken. This is a healthier version of fried chicken, and is cooked much quicker than in the oven or on the stove top.

Prep/Cook Time: 20 minutes, Servings:6, 3 SmartPoints

Ingredients

- 2 large chicken breasts
- 1 tbsp olive oil
- ½ cup (25 grams) bread crumbs
- ½ tsp paprika
- ¼ tsp dried chili powder
- ¼ tsp ground black pepper
- ¼ tsp garlic powder
- ¼ tsp onion powder
- ¼ tsp cayenne pepper
- ½ tsp salt

Instructions

- Put the chicken breasts in a bowl and drizzle with olive oil, mix the chicken to make sure that it's well coated with oil.
- In a shallow dish, mix the bread crumbs with the spices until well combined.
- Coat each chicken breast in bread crumbs, and transfer to your air fryer basket.
- Cook in the air fryer at 390F or 200C for 10-12 minutes. After the first 7 minutes, open the air fryer and flip the chicken on the other side then continue cooking (cook for 3 minutes, depending on the size of the chicken breast used).

Nutrition Info : Calories: 163kcal, Carbohydrates: 1g, Protein: 24g, Fat: 7g, Saturated Fat: 1g, Cholesterol: 72mg, Sodium: 423mg, Potassium: 418mg, Fiber: 1g, Sugar: 1g

Air Fryer Greek Stuffed Chicken Breast

Prep/Cook Time: 25 mins, 4 Servings, 3 W W FreeStyle SmartPoints

Ingredients

- 2 6-ounce boneless skinless chicken breasts
- 1 cup wild rice, prepared
- 4 ounces Fat-Free Feta Cheese
- 4 tablespoons Greek Salad Dressing

Instructions

- Slice chicken breasts in half, making a total of 4 pieces of chicken.
- Between two pieces of plastic wrap or parchment paper, pound the chicken breasts until thin.
- In a small bowl, mix together prepared wild rice, 1 tablespoon Greek dressing, and fat-free Feta cheese.
- Place ¼ rice mixture onto center of each chicken breast and roll covering mixture.
- Place each chicken breasts rolled side down into air fryer pan.
- Brush remaining Greek dressing over tops of chicken breasts
- Cook at 382 degrees for 15 minutes, or until internal temperature reaches 165 degrees.

Nutrition Info : Calories: 197kcal, Carbohydrates: 3g, Protein: 20g, Fat: 4g, Saturated Fat: 1g

The Best Air Fryer Popcorn Chicken

Prep/Cook Time: 30 minutes, Servings: 2, 3 WW smartpoints

Ingredients

- 10 ounces chicken breast, cut into bite sized pieces
- For the blackened seasoning (you won't use it all but it will store for a month)
- 1 tablespoon paprika
- 1 teaspoon white pepper
- 1 teaspoon black pepper
- 1 teaspoon salt
- 1 teaspoon cayenne pepper
- 1 teaspoon Italian seasoning
- 1 teaspoon garlic powder
- 1 teaspoon onion powder

Dipping station:
- 1 egg
- 2 tablespoons unsweetened almond milk
- 1 teaspoon hot sauce
- Flour station:
- 1/8 cup self-rising flour
- 2 teaspoons of the blackened seasoning above
- 28 grams Safe + Fair Olive Oil and Sea Salt Popcorn Quinoa Chips

Instructions

- Toss the chicken in two teaspoons of the seasoning and toss until coated.

- In a food processor* crush the popcorn quinoa chips. Mix into the flour and blackened seasoning.
- Mix the egg, almond milk and hot sauce. Dip the chicken into the egg mixture and into the popcorn quinoa flour mixture, pressing to get the batter to stick.
- Put on a paper plate and stick in the freezer for fifteen minutes. This will make sure that your batter stays on the chicken and doesn't come off on the first bite.
- Spray with avocado oil spray so that you can't see anymore flour.
- Bake in an air fryer for 6 minutes at 360, then 4-6 minutes at 400 degrees, flipping after the first 6 minutes. Depending on how big you cut your chicken, check the chicken every two minutes once you bump the heat up to 400.
- If you have a meat thermometer (and if you don't why don't you!) they are done when they reach 165 degrees.

Nutrition Info: 110 calories, Carbohydrates: 4g, Protein: 22g, Fat: 5g, Saturated Fat: 1g

Air Fryer Chicken Milanese with Arugula

Prep/Cook Time: 30 mins, 4 servings, 4 Freestyle Points

Ingredients
- 2 boneless, skinless chicken breasts, 16 oz total
- 3/4 teaspoon kosher salt
- Freshly ground black pepper
- 1/2 cup seasoned whole wheat breadcrumbs, wheat or gluten-free
- 2 tablespoons grated Parmesan cheese
- 1 large egg, beaten
- olive oil spray
- 6 cups baby arugula
- 3 lemons, cut into wedges

Instructions
- Cut chicken into 4 cutlets, then place cutlets between 2 sheets of parchment paper or plastic wrap and pound out to 1/4-inch thick.
- Sprinkle both sides with salt and pepper.
- In a shallow plate, beat the egg and 1 teaspoon of water together.
- Combine breadcrumbs and parmesan cheese in a shallow bowl.
- Dip the chicken into the egg, then the breadcrumb mixture. Place on a work surface and spray both sides with olive oil.
- Preheat the air fryer to 400F.
- In batches transfer to the air fryer basket and cook 7 minutes, turning halfway until golden and cooked through.
- Serve chicken with 1 1/2 cups arugula and top with a generous amount of lemon juice.

Oven Instructions: Bake in a preheated oven 425F 425F for 12 to 14 minutes, flipping halfway until golden.

Nutrition Info : Calories: 219kcal, Carbohydrates: 10.5g, Protein: 31g, Fat: 6g, Saturated Fat: 1.5g, Cholesterol: 131.5mg, Sodium: 563.5mg, Fiber: 1.5g, Sugar: 2g

Air Fryer Asian-Glazed Boneless Chicken Thighs

Prep/Cook Time: 2 hrs 35 mins, 4 servings, 7 Freestyle Points

Ingredients

- 32 ounces 8 boneless, skinless chicken thighs, fat trimmed
- 1/4 cup low sodium soy sauce
- 2 1/2 tablespoons balsamic vinegar
- 1 tablespoon honey
- 3 cloves garlic, crushed
- 1 teaspoon Sriracha hot sauce
- 1 teaspoon fresh grated ginger
- 1 scallion, green only sliced for garnish

Instructions

- In a small bowl combine the balsamic, soy sauce, honey, garlic, sriracha and ginger and mix well.
- Pour half of the marinade (1/4 cup) into a large bowl with the chicken, covering all the meat and marinate at least 2 hours, or as long as overnight.
- Reserve the remaining sauce for later.
- Preheat the air fryer to 400F.

- Remove the chicken from the marinade and transfer to the air fryer basket.
- Cook in batches 14 minutes, turning halfway until cooked through in the center.
- Meanwhile, place the remaining sauce in a small pot and cook over medium-low heat until it reduces slightly and thickens, about 1 to 2 minutes.
- To serve, drizzle the sauce over the chicken and top with scallions.

Nutrition Info : Calories: 297kcal, Carbohydrates: 5g, Protein: 45.5g, Fat: 9.5g, Saturated Fat: 2.5g, Cholesterol: 214mg, Sodium: 835mg, Fiber: 0.5g, Sugar: 2g

Chicken Parmesan in the Air Fryer

Prep/Cook Time: 15 mins, 4 servings, 4 Freestyle Points

Ingredients

- 2 about 8 oz each chicken breast, sliced in half to make 4 thinner cutlets
- 6 tbsp seasoned breadcrumbs, I used whole wheat, you can use gluten-free
- 2 tbsp grated Parmesan cheese
- 1 tbsp butter, melted (or olive oil)
- 6 tbsp reduced fat mozzarella cheese, I used Polly-o
- 1/2 cup marinara
- cooking spray

Instructions

- Preheat the air fryer 360F° for 3 minutes.
- Combine breadcrumbs and parmesan cheese in a bowl. Melt the butter in another bowl.

- o Lightly brush the butter onto the chicken, then dip into breadcrumb mixture.
- o When the air fryer is ready, place 2 pieces in the basket and spray the top with oil.
- o Cook 6 minutes, turn and top each with 1 tbsp sauce and 1 1/2 tbsp of shredded mozzarella cheese.
- o Cook 3 more minutes or until cheese is melted.
- o Set aside and keep warm, repeat with the remaining 2 pieces.

Nutrition Info: Calories: 251kcal, Carbohydrates: 14g, Protein: 31.5g, Fat: 9.5g, Saturated Fat:

Air-Fryer Chicken Potstickers

Prep/Cook: 30 minutes, Servings: 4, 4 Freestyle Points

Ingredients:

- 6 oz. raw lean ground chicken (at least 92% lean)
- 1/4 cup canned sliced water chestnuts, drained and chopped
- 1/4 cup chopped scallions
- 1 tbsp. dried minced onion
- 2 tsp. reduced-sodium soy sauce
- 1 1/2 tsp. seasoned rice vinegar
- 1 tsp. chopped garlic
- 1/2 tsp. ground ginger
- 16 square wonton wrappers (stocked with the tofu)
- Optional dips: sweet Asian chili sauce, additional soy sauce

Instructions:
- o In a medium bowl, combine all ingredients except wonton wrappers. Mix well.

- Lay out eight wonton wrappers on a dry surface. Top with half of the chicken mixture, about 1 tbsp. per wrapper. Moisten wrapper edges with water, and fold the bottom left corner of each wrapper to meet the top right corner, forming a triangle and enclosing the filling. Press firmly on the edges to seal. Repeat to make eight more potstickers. Spray with nonstick spray.
- Set air fryer to 392 degrees (see HG FYI). Add potstickers in a single layer. (If they won't all fit, save the remaining for a second batch.) Cook for 5 minutes, or until chicken is cooked through and wrappers are golden brown and crispy.

Nutrition Info : 152 calories, 2.5g total fat (0.5g sat fat), 323mg sodium, 20g carbs, 1g fiber, 2g sugars, 11g protein

Quick Air Fryer Tortilla Chips

Prep/Cook Time: 7 mins, Serves: 1 serving, 4 WW SmartPoints

Ingredients

- 3 extra thin corn tortillas
- Olive Oil Spray
- Salt, to taste

Instructions

- Cut each tortilla into 8 triangles. Lay flat on a baking sheet.
- Spray the triangles lightly with olive oil spray and sprinkle with salt, to taste. (Some of the salt falls off while cooking so I'm usually a little more heavy-handed than normal).

- Place triangles into the air fryer - spread the out as much as possible so the layers aren't directly on top of each other.
- Cook at 360F, shaking the basket often, for 4-5 minutes, until very crispy and just slightly brown. (Watch closely at the end because they will get brown very fast. Be sure to shake often so they don't stick together and all surfaces have a chance to get crispy). Enjoy!

Nutrition Info : Calories: 120 Fat: 2 Saturated fat: 0 Carbohydrates: 24 Sugar: 3 Fiber: 4 Protein: 3

Air Fryer Buffalo Chicken Tenders

Prep/Cook Time:30 mins, Servings: 4, 2 WW SmartPoints

Ingredients

- 1 lb. boneless skinless chicken breasts
- 1/4 c. buffalo wing sauce
- 2/3 c. Panko bread crumbs

Instructions

- Cut the chicken breasts into 1 inch thick strips. Pat the chicken dry with a paper towel.
- Pour the buffalo sauce into a small bowl. Add the Panko breadcrumbs to a seperate small bowl.
- Dip the chicken strips into the buffalo sauce and using your fingers scrape off the excess sauce. Place the dipped chicken in the bowl of Panko break crumbs and coat evenly.
- Carefully arrange the breaded chicken in your Airfryer basket. Cook at 300° for 20 minutes or the internal

temperature of the chicken reaches 165°. Serve immediately.

Nutrition Info : Calories: 285kcal, Carbohydrates: 28g, Protein: 29g, Fat: 5g, Saturated Fat: 1g, Cholesterol: 72mg, Sodium: 873mg, Potassium: 496mg

FireCracker Chicken, Slimming & W W Friendly

Prep/Cooking Time: 40 minutes, Servings 4, 2 WW Smart Points

Ingredients

- 4 medium Chicken Breasts diced, approximately 150g each
- 1/2 Red Chilli finely chopped - can leave out if you don't like chilli
- 2 Garlic Cloves finely chopped
- 1 tbsp Sweetener
- 3 tbsp Dark Soy Sauce
- 2 tbsp Oyster Sauce
- 1 tbsp Rice Vinegar
- 2 tbsp Tomato Ketchup
- 1/2 tbsp Tamarind Paste
- 1 tbsp fish sauce
- 1 grind Black Pepper
- 1 Onion sliced
- 3 Peppers sliced
- 200 g Mange Tout
- 6 Arbol Chillies any dried chillies will do or 1/2 tsp of chilli flakes
- 1 bunch spring onions chopped

- 1 wedge Limes
- 100 ml Chicken stock Made up with 1/2 stock cube and 100ml of water

Instructions
- o Add the chilli, garlic, sweetener, tomato ketchup, tamarind paste, oyster sauce, soy sauce, fish sauce and rice vinegar into a bowl. Add the black pepper to season and stir the contents of the bowl well.
- o Add the chicken breast to the bowl and mix it all together.
- o Once the chicken breasts are coated in the marinade, cover the bowl with cling film and chill in the fridge for one hour.
- o Take the bowl of marinated chicken out of fridge and place into your Actifry, and set aside the remaining marinade. Set the Actifry to cook for 10 minutes.
- o After 10 minutes is up, add the chopped onions and Frylight and set to cook for a further 5 minutes.
- o Once this is complete, add the stock, the remaining marinade, peppers, spring onions, chilli and mange tout and cook for a further 10 minutes. Once this is complete, it's ready to serve!

Nutrition Info : Calories: 157kcal, Carbohydrates: 22g, Protein: 27g, Fat: 5g

Cornflake chicken

Prep/Cook Time: 25 mins, Serves: 1, 4 Freestyle points

Ingredients

- Boneless skinless chicken breast, cut into strips
- Cornflakes
- Egg whites

Instructions

- Preheat oven to 350F, line a baking sheet with parchment paper (I like to give mine a little spray too, with cooking spray)
- Cut your chicken into strips
- Crush up your cornflakes, I like to do it the old fashioned way, in a bag and crush down with a heavy glass, then pour them out onto a plate.
- Dip your chicken pieces into the egg whites and then coat them in the cornflakes. ? cup of crushed cornflakes will coat 6oz of raw chicken, making a 5oz (cooked) serving 1 freestyle SP or 4 smart points
- Bake in oven for approx 20-25 min, turning halfway..
- Serve with your favorite dipping sauce (points not incl)

Nutrition Info : Calories: 222kcal, Carbohydrates: 13g, Protein: 7g, Fat: 9g, Saturated Fat: 1g, Cholesterol: 81mg, Sodium: 789mg, Potassium: 486mg

Air Fryer Chick-fil-A Chicken Sandwich

Prep/Cook Time: 26 minutes, Servings: 6 sandwiches

Ingredients

- 2 Chicken Breasts Boneless/Skinless pounded
- 1/2 cup Dill Pickle Juice
- 2 Eggs
- 1/2 cup Milk
- 1 cup All Purpose Flour
- 2 Tablespoons Powdered Sugar
- 2 Tablespoons Potato Starch
- 1 teaspoon Paprika
- 1 teaspoon Sea Salt
- 1/2 teaspoon Freshly Ground Black Pepper
- 1/2 teaspoon Garlic Powder
- 1/4 teaspoon Ground Celery Seed ground
- 1 Tablespoon Extra Virgin Olive Oil extra virgin
- 1 Oil Mister
- 4 Hamburger Buns toasted/buttered
- 8 Dill Pickle Chips or more

Spicy Option

- 1/4 teaspoon Cayenne Pepper for spicy sandwiches

Instructions

- Place chicken into a Ziploc Baggie and pound, so that the whole piece is the same thickness, about 1/2 inch thick. Cut chicken into two or three pieces (depending on size).

- Place pieces of chicken back into Ziploc baggie and pour in pickle juice. Marinate in the refrigerator for at least 30 minutes.
- In a medium bowl, beat egg with the milk. In another bowl, combine flour, starch and all spices.
- Using tongs, coat chicken with egg mixture and then into flour mixture, making sure pieces are completely coated. Shake off excess flour (this is important).
- Spray the basket of your air fryer with Oil and place chicken into air fryer and spray the chicken with oil.
- Cook at 340 degrees for 6 minutes. Using silicone tongs, carefully flip the chicken and spray with oil. Cook for 6 more minutes.
- Raise the temperature to 400 degrees and cook for two minutes on each side.
- Serve on buttered and toasted buns, with 2 pickle chips and a small dollop of mayonnaise, if desired.

Nutrition Info : Calories 281 Calories from Fat 54, Fat 6g, Saturated Fat 1g, Cholesterol 80mg, Sodium 984mg, Potassium 288mg, Carbohydrates 38g, Fiber 1g, Sugar 5g, Protein 15g

Air Fryer Greek Stuffed Chicken Breast

Prep/Cook Time: 25 mins, 4 Servings, 3 SmartPoints W WFreeStyle

Ingredients

- 2 6-ounce boneless skinless chicken breasts
- 1 cup wild rice, prepared
- 4 ounces Fat-Free Feta Cheese
- 4 tablespoons Greek Salad Dressing

Instructions

- Slice chicken breasts in half, making a total of 4 pieces of chicken.
- Between two pieces of plastic wrap or parchment paper, pound the chicken breasts until thin.
- In a small bowl, mix together prepared wild rice, 1 tablespoon Greek dressing, and fat-free Feta cheese.
- Place ¼ rice mixture onto center of each chicken breast and roll covering mixture.
- Place each chicken breasts rolled side down into air fryer pan.
- Brush remaining Greek dressing over tops of chicken breasts
- Cook at 382 degrees for 15 minutes, or until internal temperature reaches 165 degrees.

Nutrition Info : Calories 281 Calories from Fat 54, Fat 6g, Saturated Fat 1g, Cholesterol 80mg, Sodium 984mg, Potassium 288mg, Carbohydrates 38g, Fiber 1g, Sugar 5g, Protein 15g

Chicken schnitzel with salsa verde

Prep/Cook Time: 32 min, Serves 4, 8 SmartPoints

Ingredients

- ¼ cup(s), (35g) plain flour
- 1 medium egg(s)
- 1 cup(s), (65g) panko breadcrumbs
- ½ tsp Onion powder
- 1½ tbs olive oil
- 540 g, (4 x 150g fillets) skinless chicken breast
- 1 cup(s), (bunch) fresh flat-leaf parsley
- 1 cup(s), (bunch) fresh basil
- 80 g, (4 individual) pickled gherkin, drained
- 1 tb baby capers, rinsed, drained
- 1 tsp white wine vinegar
- 1 tbs dijon mustard
- 300 g, trimmed, halved green beans
- 500 g, halved cherry tomato

Instructions

- Place flour on a plate. Whisk egg and 2 tsp water in a shallow plate. Combine breadcrumbs, onion powder and 1 tbs oil in a third shallow plate. Season.
- Place chicken between 2 sheets of baking paper and pound with a rolling pin until an even thickness of 1.5cm. Working with 1 piece at a time, coat with flour, shaking off excess. Dip in egg and finally coat with breadcrumb mixture.
- Preheat Philips Airfryer to 200°C. Place 2 chicken pieces in Airfryer basket, taking care to allow a small

- gap between them. Place grill attachment over chicken and place remaining pieces chicken on grill. Slide basket into Airfryer. Set timer to 12 minutes. Remove from Airfryer
- Meanwhile, using a food processor, process parsley, basil, gherkins, capers, vinegar, mustard and 2 tbs water, stopping several times to scrape down side of bowl, until a rough paste forms. Season.
- Heat remaining oil in a large frying pan over high heat. Cook beans for 1 minute or until lightly charred. Season. Add tomatoes. Carefully add ¼ cup (60ml) water, standing back to avoid steam. Cook, stirring, for 1-2 minutes or until tomatoes soften slightly.
- Serve chicken schnitzel with beans and tomatoes and dollop over salsa verde.

Nutrition Info : Calories: 170kcal, Carbohydrates: 2g, Protein: 23g, Fat: 7.1g, Saturated Fat: 1g

Air Fried Chicken Philly Cheese Egg Rolls

Prep/Cook Time: 20 minutes, Servings: 8, 3 WW Freestyle SmartPoints

Ingredients
- 8 egg rolls wrappers
- 12.5 oz. canned shredded chicken or 1 1/2 cup cooked rotisserie chicken
- 1 Tbsp Worcestershire sauce
- 1/2 medium onion, diced
- 1/2 small green pepper, diced
- 4 oz. 1/3 less fat cream cheese, room temperature

Instructions
- Spray a large skillet with non stick cooking spray. Cook diced onion and green pepper over medium heat and continue cooking until the onion is clear and tender.
- Remove from heat and allow to cool.
- In a large mixing bow combine, cream cheese, Worcestershire sauce, and shredded cooked chicken. Mix until cream cheese is combined with chicken. Add onion and peppers and stir until all ingredients are well combined.
- Lay one egg roll wrapper out with a corner pointing towards you. Place about 2 Tbsp in the center of each wrapper.
- Bring the corner that is closest to you up and over and gently tuck it in. Fold in the sides and roll the wrapper tightly. Use a small amount of water to secure the tip of the wrapper.
- Repeat for all 8 wrappers.
- Place egg rolls in air fryer and cook at 390 degrees for 8-10 minutes or until the egg roll wrappers are golden brown.

Nutrition Info : Calories: 294 Total Fat: 8g Saturated Fat: 4g Trans Fat: 0g Unsaturated Fat: 12g Cholesterol: 92mg Sodium: 630mg Carbohydrates: 26g Fiber: 2g Sugar: 1g Protein: 31g

Crispy Air Fryer Chicken Tenders

Prep/Cook Time: 20 minutes, Servings: 3, 4 WW Freestyle SmartPoints

Ingredients

- 2 large chicken breasts cut into strips
- 1 tbsp olive oil
- ½ cup (25 grams) bread crumbs
- ½ tsp paprika
- ¼ tsp dried chili powder
- ¼ tsp ground black pepper
- ¼ tsp garlic powder
- ¼ tsp onion powder
- ¼ tsp cayenne pepper
- ½ tsp salt

Instructions

- Put the chicken strips in a bowl and drizzle with olive oil, mix the chicken to make sure that it's well coated with oil.
- In a shallow dish, mix the bread crumbs with the spices until well combined.
- Coat each chicken strip in bread crumbs, and transfer to your air fryer basket.
- Cook in the air fryer at 390F or 200C for 9-11 minutes. After the first 7 minutes, open the air fryer and flip the chicken on the other side then continue cooking (cook for 3 minutes, depending on the thickness the chicken used).

Nutrition Info : Calories: 163kcal, Carbohydrates: 1g, Protein: 24g, Fat: 7g, Saturated Fat: 1g, Cholesterol: 72mg, Sodium: 423mg, Potassium: 418mg

Air Fryer Chicken Tenders

Prep/Cook Time: 25 minutes, 6 W W Freestyle points

Ingredients

- 1½ lb. of Chicken Tenderloins
- Salt and pepper to taste
- 1 Egg
- 2 tablespoon of Milk
- 1 cup of all-purpose Flour
- 1 teaspoon + 1 teaspoon of Garlic Powder
- 1 teaspoon + 1 teaspoon of Paprika
- 1 cup of Panko Breadcrumbs

Instructions

- Lightly season the chicken tenders with salt and pepper.
- Crack the egg in a bowl. Add the milk, salt and pepper and whisk it well.
- In a shallow bowl, combine the flour, salt and pepper, 1 teaspoon of garlic powder and 1 teaspoon of paprika. Mix it well.
- In another shallow bowl combine the panko breadcrumbs, salt and pepper, 1 teaspoon of garlic powder and 1 teaspoon of paprika. Mix it well.
- Take a chicken tender. Dredge it in the all-purpose flour mix. Shake off the excess. Dip it in the egg mix. And then coat it completely with the panko breadcrumb mix. Keep it aside on a wire rack.
- Repeat with all the chicken tenders.

- Place few slices in the lightly greased air fryer basket, in a single layer. Lightly spray the crumb coated tenders.
- Air fry at 370 F for 14 minutes, flipping at the halfway mark (at 7 minutes).
- Repeat with all the prepared chicken tenders.
- Serve hot with ketchup or ranch.

Nutrition Info

Calories: 201kcal, Carbohydrates: 4g, Protein: 25g, Fat: 8g, Saturated Fat: 4g, Cholesterol: 8mg, Sodium: 432mg, Potassium: 501mg

WW AIRFRYER BEEF & PORK RECIPES

Prep/Cook Time: 15 mins, Servings : 6, 7 W W Freestyle points

Ingredients

- olive oil spray
- 6 3/4-inch thick center cut boneless pork chops, fat trimmed (5 oz each)
- kosher salt
- 1 large egg, beaten
- 1/2 cup panko crumbs, check labels for GF
- 1/3 cup crushed cornflakes crumbs
- 2 tbsp grated parmesan cheese, omit for dairy free
- 1 1/4 tsp sweet paprika
- 1/2 tsp garlic powder
- 1/2 tsp onion powder
- 1/4 tsp chili powder
- 1/8 tsp black pepper

Instructions

- Preheat the air fryer to 400F for 12 minutes and lightly spray the basket with oil.
- Season pork chops on both sides with 1/2 tsp kosher salt.
- Combine panko, cornflake crumbs, parmesan cheese, 3/4 tsp kosher salt, paprika, garlic powder, onion powder, chili powder and black pepper in a large shallow bowl.
- Place the beaten egg in another. Dip the pork into the egg, then crumb mixture.
- When the air fryer is ready, place 3 of the chops into the prepared basket and spritz the top with oil.
- Cook 12 minutes turning half way, spritzing both sides with oil. Set aside and repeat with the remaining.

Nutrition Info : Serving: 1pork chop, Calories: 378kcal, Carbohydrates: 8g, Protein: 33g, Fat: 13g, Cholesterol: 121mg, Sodium: 373mg, Sugar: 1g

Air Fryer Beef Empanadas

Prep/Cook Time: 30 mins, 8 servings, 5 W W Freestyle points

Ingredients

- 8 Goya empanada discs, in frozen section, thawed
- 1 cup picadillo
- 1 egg white, whisked
- 1 teaspoon water

Instructions

- Preheat the air fryer to 325F for 8 minutes. Spray the basket generously with cooking spray.
- Place 2 tbsp of picadillo in the center of each disc. Fold in half and use a fork to seal the edges. Repeat with the remaining dough.
- Whisk the egg whites with water, then brush the tops of the empanadas.
- Bake 2 or 3 at a time in the air fryer 8 minutes, or until golden. Remove from heat and repeat with the remaining empanadas.

Nutrition Info : Calories: 183kcal, Carbohydrates: 22g, Protein: 11g, Fat: 5g, Saturated Fat: 1g, Cholesterol: 16mg, Sodium: 196mg, Fiber: 1g, Sugar: 2.5g

That Man's Pork Chops

Total 25 mins, Servings 4, 3 oz Servings, 3 W WFreesty

Ingredients

- 4 lean boneless pork chops (approximately 3 oz each)
- 1 Tbsp Nutritional Yeast
- 1 tsp favorite seasoning (I use Dak's Red Mountain Rub)
- olive oil non stick spray

Instructions

- Lightly spray each pork chop with non stick spray.
- Sprinkle evenly with the nutritional yeast and seasoning. Place in Simple Living Products Air Fryer basket in a single layer.
- Change settings to 360 and 20 minutes and start. Normal boneless pork chops are so thin there is no need to flip!
- Check with a meat thermometer and serve while hot. Deliciously "fried"!

Nutrition Info : Calories: 147kcal, Carbohydrates: 3g, Protein: 9g, Fat: 11g, Saturated Fat: 6g, Cholesterol: 188mg, Sodium: 133mg, Potassium: 237mg, Fiber: 1g, Sugar: 1g

Beef and Vegetables Stir Fry with Noodles

Prep/Cook Time: 20 min, Servings: 4, 3 W W Freestyle points

Ingredients

- 400 g 14 oz rump steak cut 1.5 cm thick
- 2 ActiFry spoons of toasted sesame oil
- 600 g 1lb 5 oz stir fry vegetables
- 6 tablespoons hoisin sauce
- 250 g 9 oz fine egg noodles, cooked

Instructions

- Trim excess fat off the beef and cut into thin strips (6mm thick). Add 1 ActiFry spoonful of sesame oil and heat for 2 minutes in the ActifFy, Cook the beef for 5 minutes or until still pink in the centre (it will finish cooking in step 3). If the meat clumps together, half way through cooking break apart with a fork. Remove beef to a plate: set aside and keep warm.
- Add stir fry vegetables and drizzle over 1 ActiFry spoonful of sesame oil. Cook for 5 minutes or until vegetables are cooked and still crunchy.
- In a bowl, mix together the hoisin sauce and 2 tablespoons of water; add to the vegetables together with the beef. Stir well with a wooden spoon. Cook for 3-4 minutes or until hot. Serve with cooked fine egg noodles.

Nutrition Info : Calories: 156kcal, Carbohydrates: 2g, Protein: 8g, Fat: 16g

Beef and Broccoli Stir-Fry

Prep/Cook Time: 28 min, Serves 4, 3 W W Smartpoints

Ingredients

- 2½ Tbsp, divided cornstarch
- ¼ tsp table salt
- ¾ pound(s), thinly sliced against the grain uncooked lean trimmed sirloin beef
- 2 tsp canola oil
- 1 cup(s), divided reduced-sodium chicken broth
- 5 cup(s), florets (about a 12 oz bag) uncooked broccoli
- 1 Tbsp, fresh, minced ginger root
- 2 tsp minced garlic
- ¼ tsp, or to taste red pepper flakes
- ¼ cup(s) water
- ¼ cup(s) low sodium soy sauce

Instructions

- On a plate, combine 2 tablespoons cornstarch and salt; add beef and toss to coat.
- Heat oil in a large nonstick wok or large deep skillet over medium-high heat. Add beef and stir-fry until lightly browned and cooked through, about 4 minutes; transfer to a bowl with a slotted spoon.
- Add 1/2 cup broth to same pan; stir to loosen any bits on food on bottom of pan. Add broccoli; cover and cook, tossing occasionally and sprinkling with a tablespoon water if needed, until broccoli is almost crisp-tender, about 3 minutes. Uncover pan and add

- ginger, garlic and red pepper flakes; stir-fry until fragrant, about 1 minute.
  o In a cup, stir together water, soy sauce, remaining 1/2 cup broth and remaining 1/2 tablespoon cornstarch until blended; stir into pan. Reduce heat to medium-low and bring to a simmer; simmer until slightly thickened, about 1 minute.
  o Return beef and accumulated juices to pan; toss to coat. Serve. Servings s about 1 1/4 cups per serving.

Nutrition Info: Calories: 188kcal, Carbohydrates: 4g, Protein: 8g, Fat: 17g, Saturated Fat: 7g, Cholesterol: 198mg, Sodium: 143mg, Potassium: 433mg

Ww Oven-Fried Pork Chops 5-Points

Prep/Cook Time: 1hr 5mins, Serves: 4, 5 W W Freestyle Points

Ingredients

- 4 (6 ounce) center-cut pork loin chops, lean
- 2 tablespoons pineapple juice
- 1 tablespoon low sodium soy sauce
- 1/4 teaspoon ground ginger
- 1/8 teaspoon garlic powder
- 1 large egg white, lightly beaten
- 1/3 cup dry breadcrumbs
- 1/4 teaspoon dried Italian seasoning
- 1/4 teaspoon paprika
- 1 dash garlic powder
- cooking spray

Instructions

- Preheat oven to 350 degrees.
- Trim fat from chops.
- Combine juice and next 4 ingredients in a bowl; stir well.
- Combine breadcrumbs, Italian seasoning, paprika, and dash of garlic powder in a shallow dish; stir well.
- Dip chops in juice mixture, and dredge in breadcrumbs mixture.
- Place chops on a broiler pan coated with cooking spray.
- Bake at 350 degrees for 50 minutes or until tender, turning after 25 minutes.

Nutrition Info : Calories 291 Fat 8g Satfat 4g Unsatfat 3g Protein 17g Carbohydrate 36g Fiber 8g Sugars 3g Added sugars 0g Sodium 518mg

Barbecued Pork Chops

Prep/Cook Time:20 minutes, 4 Servings, Freestyle SmartPoints: 8

Ingredients

- 1/4 cup packed brown sugar
- 1/4 cup ketchup
- 1 Tablespoon worcestershire sauce
- 1 Tablespoon low-sodium soy sauce
- 1 teaspoon dried thyme
- 1 teaspoon garlic salt
- 1/4 teaspoon ground red pepper
- 4 whole boneless loin chops (about 1 1/2 pounds total)

Instructions

- Preheat grill or broiler.
- Combine first 4 ingredients in a small bowl. Remove 1/4 cup of the sauce to a small bowl and set aside.
- Combine thyme, garlic salt and red pepper; sprinkle over one side of the chops. Place the chops on a grill rack or broiler pan coated with cooking spray; cook 5 to 6 minutes per side, basting with the remaining sauce. After cooking, let rest 5 minutes. Serve with remaining sauce (heated).

Nutrition Info : Calories: 274, Fat: 4g, Saturated Fat: 1.23g, Sugar: 16.64g, Sodium: 1184mg, Fiber: .5g, Protein: 39g, Cholesterol: 94mg, Carbohydrates: 19g

Pork Cacciatore

Prep/Cook Time: 44 min, Serves 4, Freestyle SmartPoints: 3

Ingredients

- 3 spray(s), divided cooking spray
- 12 oz, cut into 1- to 1 1/2-in chunks uncooked lean pork tenderloin
- ½ tsp, divided table salt
- ½ tsp, freshly ground, divided black pepper
- 3 small, peeled, cut into 1-in chunks uncooked Yukon gold potato(es)
- 1 medium, halved and thinly sliced uncooked onion(s)
- ¾ cup(s), or more if necessary, divided water
- 1 medium, cut into 1-in chunks yellow pepper(s)

- 8 oz, halved or quartered lengthwise (about 3 cups) cremini mushroom(s)
- ¾ tsp, or to taste dried rosemary
- 1 cup(s) store bought marinara sauce

Instructions

- Coat a large nonstick skillet with cooking spray; heat over medium heat. Sprinkle pork with 1/4 teaspoon each salt and pepper. Add pork to skillet, increase heat to medium-high and cook, turning pieces occasionally, until browned, about 6 minutes; remove to a plate.
- Off heat, coat same skillet with cooking spray; heat over medium heat. Add potatoes, onion and 1/2 cup of water; cook, scraping bottom of pan, 1 minute. Cover and cook, stirring occasionally, 5 minutes.
- Add yellow pepper, mushrooms, rosemary and remaining 1/4 teaspoon each salt and pepper to skillet; sauté over medium-high heat, until vegetables are lightly browned, adding a tablespoon or two of water if needed to prevent sticking, about 7 minutes.
- Stir in marinara sauce, pork and 1/4 cup water; bring to a simmer. Cover skillet, reduce heat to medium and cook until vegetables are tender and pork is cooked through, about 7 minutes. Servings s about 1 1/2 cups per serving.

Nutrition Info : Calories: 222, Fat: 8g, Saturated Fat: 2g, Sugar: 17g, Sodium: 904mg, Fiber: 0.5g, Protein: 41g

Air-fried Burgers

Prep/Cook Time: 20 minutes, Servings 4, 4 W WFreestyle points

Ingredients

- 1 Tablespoon Worcestershire sauce
- 1 teaspoon Maggi seasoning sauce
- liquid smoke (few drops)
- 1/2 teaspoon garlic powder
- 1/2 teaspoon onion powder
- 1/2 teaspoon salt (or salt sub)
- 1/2 teaspoon ground black pepper
- 1 teaspoon parsley (dried)
- 500 g ground beef (Raw. 1 lb.)

Instructions

- Spray the upper Actifry tray; set aside. If you are using a basket-type fryer, no need to spray the basket. In basket-types, your cooking temperature will be 180 C / 350 F.
- In a small bowl, mix together all the seasoning items, from the Worcestershire sauce down to and including the dried parsley.
- Add this to the beef in a large bowl.
- Mix well, but be careful not to overwork the meat as that leads to tough burgers.
- Divide the beef mixture into 4, and shape the patties. With your thumb, put an indent in the centre of each one to prevent the patties bunching up in the middle.
- Put tray in Actifry; spray tops of patties lightly.
- Cook 10 minutes for medium (or longer to desired degree of doneness). There is no need to turn the patties.
- Serve hot on a bun with side dishes of your choice.

Nutrition Info : Serving: 1g, Calories: 148kcal, Protein: 24.2g, Fat: 4.6g

Crispy Breaded Pork Chops in the Air Fryer

Prep/Cook Time: 15 mins, Servings : 6, 7 W WFreestyle points

Ingredients

- olive oil spray
- 6 3/4-inch thick center cut boneless pork chops, fat trimmed (5 oz each)
- kosher salt
- 1 large egg, beaten
- 1/2 cup panko crumbs, check labels for GF
- 1/3 cup crushed cornflakes crumbs
- 2 tbsp grated parmesan cheese, omit for dairy free
- 1 1/4 tsp sweet paprika
- 1/2 tsp garlic powder
- 1/2 tsp onion powder
- 1/4 tsp chili powder
- 1/8 tsp black pepper

Instructions

- Preheat the air fryer to 400F for 12 minutes and lightly spray the basket with oil.
- Season pork chops on both sides with 1/2 tsp kosher salt.
- Combine panko, cornflake crumbs, parmesan cheese, 3/4 tsp kosher salt, paprika, garlic powder, onion powder, chili powder and black pepper in a large shallow bowl.
- Place the beaten egg in another. Dip the pork into the egg, then crumb mixture.

- When the air fryer is ready, place 3 of the chops into the prepared basket and spritz the top with oil.
- Cook 12 minutes turning half way, spritzing both sides with oil. Set aside and repeat with the remaining.

Nutrition Info : Calories: 378kcal, Carbohydrates: 8g, Protein: 33g, Fat: 13g, Cholesterol: 121mg, Sodium: 373mg, Sugar: 1g

WW AIRFRYER SOUPS AND STEWS RECIPES

Healthy & Quick W W Instant Pot Chicken Noodle Soup

Prep/Cook Time: 22 mins, Serves: 4-6, 8 W W Freestyle points

Ingredients
- 1 Large White Onion, Chopped Small
- 2 Celery Stalks, Chopped Small
- 4 Carrots, Peeled and Sliced in Rounds or Diagonally
- Salt & White Pepper to Taste
- 6 Cups of Fat Free Chicken Broth
- 2 Cups of Cooked Skinless & Boneless Chicken Breast, Shredded or Diced
- 2 Cups of Cooked Egg Noodles (Keep separate)
- Butter Flavored Cooking Spray
- Fresh Parsley, Snipped, Optional

Instructions
- Spray the base of the Instant Pot with butter flavored vegetable spray, set on saute mode and turn on to heat. Add in 3 tablespoons of water along with the onion and cook for about 2 minutes. Now add in the celery and carrots and continue cooking for 5 minutes.
- Add in the cooked chicken and the broth. Season to taste with salt and pepper.
- Cover the Instant Pot and cook on the the Soup setting for 5 minutes.
- Release pressure, uncover the Instant Pot and stir together well. Add in more salt and/or pepper to taste.
- If serving immediately, put ½ cup of cooked egg noodles into 4 bowls, add soup and enjoy. Top with fresh snipped parsley, if using. If freezing, divide the cooked egg noodles among 4 containers, add soup, cool and freeze.
- This makes 4 servings at 3 Points per serving or you can spread this out to 6 servings. Just place ? cup of

noodles into each bowl. Doing this will change the points from 3 to 2 per serving.

Nutrition Info : Calories: 121, Total Fat: 4g, Saturated Fat: 1g, Protein: 9g

Weight Watchers Zero Point Asian Soup Recipe

Prep/Cook Time: 20 minutes, Servings: 8, 4 W W Freestyle points

Ingredients

- 2 cups bok choy, chopped
- 2 cups Napa cabbage, chopped
- 5 cloves garlic, minced
- 1/4 cup fresh ginger root, thinly sliced and julienned
- 6 ounces. shitake mushrooms, sliced
- 2 cups scallions, chopped
- 1 cup canned water chestnuts, sliced (8 oz can)
- 1 can bamboo shoots, sliced (5 oz. can)
- 1/2 cup red bell pepper, thinly sliced
- 1/4 teaspoon red pepper flakes
- 8 cups vegetable broth
- 1 cup fresh bean sprouts or half of 1 can of bean sprouts, optional
- 2 cups snow peas, stringed
- 2 Tablespoons low-sodium soy sauce
- 1/2 cup cilantro, finely chopped

Instructions

o Put boc choy, Napa cabbage, garlic, ginger root, shitake mushrooms, scallions, water chestnuts, bamboo shoots, red bell pepper, pepper flakes and vegetable stock into a large soup pot. Stir to combine. Cover and bring to a boil over high heat. Reduce heat to low and simmer, partally covered for approximtely 10 minutes.

- Add bean sprouts, if using, soy sauce and snow peas. Cook for an additional 4 minutes. Stir in cilantro and serve piping hot.
- Enjoy!

Nutrition Info : Calories: 84 Total Fat: 1g Saturated Fat: 0g Trans Fat: 0g Unsaturated Fat: 0g Cholesterol: 0mg Sodium: 837mg Carbohydrates: 16g Net Carbohydrates: 0g Fiber: 4g Sugar: 7g Sugar Alcohols: 0g Protein: 6g

Greek Orzo and Chicken Soup

Prep/Cook Time: 40 minutes, Servings 4 s (2 cups per serving), WW Freestyle SmartPoints: 3

Ingredients

- 6 cups fat-free, low-sodium chicken broth
- 1 teaspoon finely chopped fresh dill
- 1 cup uncooked orzo pasta (or can sub cauliflower rice)
- 4 large eggs
- 1/3 cup freshly squeezed lemon juice
- 1 cup shredded carrot
- 1/4 teaspoon salt
- 1/4 teaspoon pepper
- 8 ounces roasted chicken breast

Instructions

- Bring the broth and dill to a boil in a large saucepan. Add the orzo. Reduce the heat, and simmer 5 minutes or until the orzo is slightly tender. Remove from heat.
- Place the eggs and juice in a blender; process until smooth. Remove 1 cup of broth from the pan with a ladle, making sure to leave out the orzo. With the blender on, slowly add the broth; process until smooth.
- Add the carrot, salt, pepper and chicken to the pan. Bring to a simmer over medium-low heat, and cook 5 minutes or until the orzo is tender. Reduce the heat to

low. Slowly stir in the egg mixture; cook 30 seconds, stirring constantly (do not boil).

Nutrition Info : Calories 345 Calories from Fat 72, Fat 8g, Saturated Fat 2g, Cholesterol 259mg, Sodium 1685mg, Potassium 532mg, Carbohydrates 33g, Fiber 2g, Sugar 3g, Protein 31g

Whole Wheat Orzo, Cauliflower & Kale Soup

Prep/Cook Time: 35 minutes, Servings: 4 Servings, 4 W W Freestyle SP

Ingredients
- 2 teaspoons olive oil
- 1 onion chopped
- 1 carrot diced
- 1 celery stalk diced
- 3 garlic cloves minced
- 1/2 teaspoon dried thyme
- 1/2 teaspoon crushed dried rosemary
- 1/2 teaspoon red pepper flakes
- 1/4 teaspoon ground pepper
- 2 tablespoons tomato paste
- 2 cups small cauliflower florets about 1/2 pound
- 7 cups low sodium vegetable broth
- 2/3 cup whole wheat orzo pasta
- 4 cups chopped kale leaves
- salt to taste*

Instructions
- Heat the olive oil in a large saucepan set over medium heat. Add the onion, carrot and celery, and cook until the vegetables are beginning to soften, about 5 minutes.
- Stir in the garlic, thyme, rosemary, red pepper flakes, salt and pepper, and cook for 1 minute. Stir in the tomato paste and cook for 1 minute.

- Add the cauliflower florets and vegetable broth, and bring to a boil over medium-high heat. Reduce to a simmer and cook for 5 minutes.
- Increase the heat to medium-high and stir in the orzo. Cook until the pasta is almost al dente.
- Stir in the kale and cook until just wilted, about 1 minute. Serve.

Nutrition Info : Calories: 203.8kcal, Carbohydrates: 39.9g, Protein: 6.8g, Fat: 2.4g, Saturated Fat: 0.2g, Sodium: 369.7mg, Fiber: 9g, Sugar: 9.2g

Spaghetti & Meatball Soup

Servings : 6 (1-1/2 cup) servings, 6 Weight Watchers Freestyle SP

Ingredients:

- 6 oz extra lean (99% lean) ground turkey (or chicken) breast
- 1/8 teaspoon garlic powder
- 1 tablespoon grated Parmesan
- 2 tablespoons plain breadcrumbs
- 1 ¼ teaspoon Italian seasoning, divided
- 1 egg white
- 1 tablespoon skim milk
- 1 tablespoon olive oil, divided
- 2 medium carrots, grated (I used a box grater)
- 1 small zucchini, grated (I used a box grater)
- ½ medium onion, diced small
- 2 garlic cloves, minced
- Salt & pepper
- 32 oz fat free, reduced sodium chicken broth
- 24 oz jar of marinara sauce

- ¼ teaspoon crushed red pepper flakes
- 1 cup uncooked broken wheat spaghetti pieces (1 inch sticks)
- 1 oz Parmesan cheese, freshly grated

Instructions

- In a large bowl, combine the ground turkey, garlic powder, tablespoon of grated Parmesan, breadcrumbs, ¾ teaspoon of the Italian seasoning, egg white and milk. Using your hands (or a spoon), mush all the ingredients together until well combined. Roll meat mixture into 30 separate (3/4" – 1") mini meatballs.
- In a large stock pot (or a large skillet, which is what I used before realizing you could totally use one pot for the entire meal and have one less to wash!), bring 2 teaspoons of the olive oil over medium heat. Add the meatballs to the oil and cook them, stirring occasionally until all sides are browned. Remove meatballs to a dish and set aside.
- Add the remaining teaspoon of olive oil to the pot and continue to heat to medium. Add the carrots, zucchini, onion and garlic and sprinkle with salt & pepper. Cook for about 5 minutes or until vegetables are softened.
- Add the meatballs, chicken broth, marinara sauce, red pepper flakes and remaining ½ teaspoon of Italian seasoning to the pot with the vegetables. Stir together and cover. Bring the mixture to a boil, uncover and lower the heat to a simmer. Add the spaghetti pieces and simmer for 12-15 minutes or until the pasta and the meatballs are cooked through. Add the Parmesan cheese in the last couple minutes of the simmer and stir in.

Nutrition Info : 244 calories, 30 g carbs, 9 g sugars, 7 g fat, 2 g saturated fat, 18 g protein, 5 g fiber

Smoked Ham Soup with White Beans

Prep/Cook Time:1 hour and 50 minutes, 8 servings, 6 W W Freestyle SP

Ingredients

- 1 tablespoon olive oil
- 1 large yellow onion, chopped
- 4 cloves garlic, minced
- 6 cups fat-free, low sodium chicken broth
- 2 cups water
- 2 tablespoons chopped fresh parsley
- 1 teaspoon chopped fresh thyme
- 1/4 teaspoon salt
- 1/4 teaspoon freshly ground black pepper
- Two 14.5-ounce cans white beans, drained & rinsed
- 2 bay leaves
- ham hock, optional
- 2 cups chopped smoked ham
- One 14.5-ounce can petite diced tomatoes, undrained

Instructions

- Heat oil in pan over medium heat. Add onion and sauté until tender, stirring occasionally. Add garlic, and cook for 1 minute, stirring frequently. Add broth, water, parsley, thyme, salt, pepper and bay leaves. If you happen to have a ham hock available to you, throw that in too. Bring to a boil. Cover and reduce heat; simmer for about an hour.
- Add beans and simmer for an additional 10 minutes. Discard bay leaves. Remove ham hock (if using).

o Place 1 cup of bean mixture in a blender or food processor; process until smooth. Return pureed bean mixture to the pan, add chopped ham and tomatoes and stir until blended. Simmer for about 5 minutes, until ham is heated through, and then serve.

Nutrition Info : Calories: 235, Fat: 4.21g, Saturated Fat: 1g, Sugar: 2g, Sodium: 985g, Fiber: 6.67g, Protein: 18.72g, Cholesterol: 19.25mg, Carbohydrates: 31.34g

Italian Vegetable Soup

Prep/Cook Time: 1 hour, Servings 8 servings, 4 W W Freestyle SP

Ingredients

- 2 teaspoons olive oil
- 1 medium sweet onion, chopped
- 2 teaspoons chopped fresh oregano
- 4 medium garlic cloves, minced
- 3 cups peeled, seeded & chopped butternut or acorn squash
- 3 cups chopped zucchini (about 4 medium)
- 1 cup fresh or frozen corn kernels
- 2 14.5-ounce cans petite diced tomatoes, drained
- 3 14-ounce cans fat-free low-sodium chicken or vegetable broth
- 1 15.5-ounce can white beans, drained & rinsed
- 1 bunch cleaned & chopped Swiss chard (leaves only... leave out the ribs)
- 1 teaspoon sea salt
- 1/2 teaspoon freshly ground black pepper

- 1/2 cup freshly grated Parmesan cheese

Instructions

- Heat the oil in a large pot over medium-high heat. Add the onion to the pot and sauté for a couple of minutes, until softened a bit. Add the oregano and garlic; sauté 1 minute. Stir in the squash, zucchini and corn, and continue to sauté a few more minutes until veggies begin to get tender. Remove from heat.
- Place 1 can of (drained) tomatoes and 1 can of broth in a blender and process until smooth. Pour into the pot with the vegetables and return to heat. Stir in the second can of (drained) tomatoes and 2 cans of broth. Bring the mixture to a boil; reduce heat and simmer for about 20 minutes.
- Add the beans and Swiss chard to the pot and stir until the chard begins to wilt (about 5 minutes). Remove from heat and stir in salt and pepper.
- Ladle the soup into bowls and sprinkle Parmesan on top of each individual serving.

Nutrition Info : Calories 188 Calories from Fat 27, Fat 3g, Saturated Fat 1g, Cholesterol 5mg, Sodium 1148mg, Potassium 919mg, Carbohydrates 30g, Fiber 6g, Sugar 5g, Protein 11g

Chicken Vegetable Soup Recipe

Prep/Cook Time:7 hrs 20 mins, Servings (adjustable): 10, Weight Watchers Freestyle SmartPoints: 0

Ingredients

- 1-1/2 pounds raw boneless skinless lean chicken breasts
- 1/2 teaspoon salt
- 1/8 teaspoon black pepper
- 1/2 cup finely diced onion
- 2 carrots, chopped
- 3 cups dry coleslaw mix (shredded cabbage and carrots)
- 2 cans (14 to 15 ounces each) low-sodium chicken broth
- 1 can (14 to 15 ounces) cannellini (white kidney) beans, drained and rinsed
- 1 can (14 to 15 ounces) stewed tomatoes, not drained
- 1 cup frozen peas
- 1 teaspoon dried thyme leaves
- 1 bay leaf

Instructions
- Ideal slow cooker size: 6-Quart.
- Evenly season chicken with 1/4 teaspoon salt and the pepper. Place all ingredients in the crock pot and stir.
- Cover and cook on HIGH for 3 to 4 hours, or on LOW for 6 - 8 hours, until chicken is fully cooked and the vegetables are tender.
- Remove and discard the bay leaf.
- Remove the chicken and place in a bowl. Shred each piece using two forks -- one to hold the chicken in place and the other to scrape across the meat and shred it.
- Return the shredded chicken to the crock pot and stir into the soup.
- Season to taste with salt and pepper.

Nutrition Info : Calories 150 Calories from Fat 9, Fat 1g, Carbohydrates 15g, Fiber 4g, Protein 20g

Zucchini and Rosemary Soup

Prep/Cook Time: 1 hour 10 min, 8 servings, W Wa Freestyle SmartPoints: 3

Ingredients

- 2 tablespoons butter
- 1 tablespoon vegetable oil
- 1 large onion, chopped
- 2 cloves garlic, sliced
- 2 teaspoons minced fresh rosemary
- 4 cups low-sodium, fat free chicken or vegetable broth
- 1 medium russet potato, peeled & sliced
- 3 medium zucchini, thinly sliced
- 1 medium zucchini, cut into 1/2-inch cubes
- green onions for topping, optional

Instructions

- Heat the butter with the oil in heavy large saucepan over medium-high heat. Add the onion; sauté until translucent, about 5 minutes. Mix in the garlic and rosemary. Add the broth and potato; bring to boil. Reduce heat and simmer 10 minutes. Add the sliced zucchini; simmer until tender, about 15 minutes. Working in batches, puree in blender. Season with salt and pepper.
- Cook the cubed zucchini in saucepan of boiling salted water for 30 seconds. Drain. Rewarm soup over medium heat. Ladle into bowls. Top with the cubed zucchini. Sprinkle with green onions.

Nutrition Info: Calories 89, Fat 5g, Saturated Fat 2g, Sugar 2.5g, Fiber 2g, Protein 2.5g, Cholesterol 8mg, Carbohydrates 10g

Slow Cooker Potato Soup for Weight Watchers

Prep/Cooking time 2 hours 10mins, 10 servings, SmartPoints: 3.5

Ingredients

- 1 (26 to 30-ounce) bag frozen hash browns
- 2 (14-ounce) cans non-fat chicken broth
- 1 (10.75-ounce) can 98% fat-free cream of chicken soup
- 1/4 cup onion, chopped
- 1/4 teaspoon black pepper
- 1 (8-ounce) package low-fat cream cheese
- 1 cup fat-free milk
- Green onions, chopped, to garnish
- Bacon bits, optional, to garnish

Instructions

- Add hash browns, chicken broth, chicken soup, onion, and black pepper to your slow-cooker and cook on high for an hour. Stir, then turn your slow-cooker to low for another hour.
- Add cream cheese, and cook another 1/2 hour or until cheese can be stirred into the mixture.
- Add milk and cook 10 to 15 minutes longer.
- Garnish with chopped green onion and bacon bits. Add 1 WW point for garnish.

Nutrition Info : Calories 100, Fat 6g, Saturated Fat 3g, Sugar 4g, Fiber 3g, Protein 5g, Cholesterol 7mg, Carbohydrates 12g

WW AIRFRYER DESSERTS RECIPES

Air Fryer Baked Potato Recipe - Baked Garlic Parsley Potatoes

Prep/Cook Time: 40 minutes, Servings: 3, 6 WWFreestyle SmartPoints

Ingredients

- 3 Idaho or Russet Baking Potatoes
- 1-2 Tablespoons Olive Oil
- 1 Tablespoon Salt
- 1 Tablespoon Garlic
- 1 Teaspoon Parsley

Instructions

- Wash your potatoes and then create air holes with a fork in the potatoes.
- Sprinkle them with the olive oil & seasonings, then rub the seasoning evenly on the potatoes.
- Once the potatoes are coated place them into the basket for the Air Fryer and place into the machine.
- Cook your potatoes at 392 degrees for 35-40 minutes or until fork tender.
- Top with your favorites. We love fresh parsley and sour cream!

Nutrition Info : Calories: 213kcal, Carbohydrates: 39g, Protein: 4g, Fat: 4g, Sodium: 2336mg, Potassium: 888mg, Fiber: 2g, Sugar: 1g, Vitamin C: 13mg, Calcium: 33mg, Iron: 1.8mg

Air Fryer Chickpea Tacos

Prep/Cook Time:15 mins, Servings: 4, 4 W WFreestyle SmartPoints

Ingredients

- 14 oz 400g tin rinsed and drained and dried
- 2 tsp olive oil
- ½ tsp smoked paprika
- ½ ground cumin
- Salt
- 8 small corn tortillas
- Taco toppings
- Radishes thinly sliced
- Avocado
- Shredded cabbage
- Cranberries
- Coconut yoghurt
- Lime

Instructions

- Pre heat air fryer to 390F / 200C.
- Mix all the ingredients together in a bowl.
- Add the chickpeas in to the air fryer basket.
- Cook for 12-15 mins turning half way through.
- Assemble tacos and top with coconut yoghurt and limes for squeezing.

Nutrition Info : Calories: 133kcal, Carbohydrates: 23g, Protein: 2g, Fat: 3g, Sodium: 23mg, Potassium: 96mg, Fiber: 3g, Calcium: 42mg, Iron: 0.6mg

2 Ingredient Dough Cinnamon Rolls

Prep/Cook Time:30 mins, Servings: 24 rolls, 4 W W Freestyle SmartPoints

Ingredients

- 1 cup nonfat Greek yogurt (Fage is best)
- 1 cup self-rising flour
- 1/4 teaspoon vanilla bean paste (see notes)
- 1/4 teaspoon cinnamon
- for icing:
- 1/2 cup whipped cream cheese
- 1/2 teaspoon cinnamon
- 1/2 teaspoon splenda, water

Instructions

- Combine yogurt, flour, vanilla bean paste, and cinnamon together in a mixing bowl. Knead by hand until the dough forms a ball. Roll out onto floured surface.
- Combine cream cheese, cinnamon, Splenda, and a few teaspoons water. Using picture as reference, roll out dough into three sections. Cut each section into 8 pieces. You will get 24 rolls total.
- Place in Air Fryer at 400*F for about 12 minutes. You can also bake these in the oven.
- Once you remove the cinnamon rolls from the Air Fryer, drizzle with remaining cream cheese mixture. You may need to heat it up a bit to make it thin enough to drizzle.

Nutrition Info: Calories: 134kcal, Carbohydrates: 19g, Protein: 2.1g, Fat: 5g

Air Fryer Monkey Bread

Prep/Cook Time: 14 mins, Servings: 8, 5 W W Freestyle SmartPoints

Ingredients
- 1 cup self rising flour
- 1 cup non-fat greek yogurt
- 1 teaspoon of sugar
- 1/2 teaspoon cinnamon

Instructions
- In a bowl, mix yogurt and self rising flour. It'll appear crumbly at first, but keep going and the dough will form.
- Make a round ball of dough out of it. Then cut into 4ths.
- Take a wedge of dough and form a flattened circular disc (as shown in previous photo). Cut into 8 pieces (like a pizza). Take each wedge and roll into balls.
- Add cinnamon and sugar into a plastic ziploc bag, and then add your balls of dough. Seal the bag and shake well to evenly coat them.
- Light spray a mini loaf pan with non-stick spray. Add your dough balls, and sprinkle just a little bit of the cinnamon sugar mix on top. i used just a pinch as there was still a lot left in the bag unused.
- Place mini loaf pan in air fryer and bake for 7 minutes at 375 degrees F.
- Allow to cool for a couple of minutes and enjoy!

Nutrition Info: Calories: 133kcal, Carbohydrates: 23g, Protein: 2g, Fat: 3g, Sodium: 23mg, Potassium: 96mg, Fiber: 3g, Calcium: 42mg, Iron: 0.6mg

Weight Watchers Air Fryer Empanadas

Prep/Cook Time: 14 mins, Servings: 8, 3 W WFreestyle SmartPoints

Ingredients

- 1 cup nonfat Greek yogurt
- 1 cup self-rising flour, divided
- 2 teaspoons garlic powder
- 1 cup cooked protein of choice (see notes)
- 1/2 cup corn , 1/4 cup salsa
- pinch of salt , eggwash

Instructions

- Combine nonfat Greek yogurt plus 3/4 self-rising flour and 2 teaspoons garlic powder.
- Roll out onto floured surface using the other 1/4 cup flour.
- Cut dough into 4 equal pieces. Roll out thin.
- Fill each section of dough with cooked meat (see notes), corn, salsa, and salt.
- Fold over, press edges with fork, eggwash (see notes)
- Preheat Air Fryer at 325*. Spray Air Fryer with noncook spray.
- Cook 1 empanada at a time in Air Fryer at 325* for 8-10 minutes. Flip over and cook for another 5-7 minutes. (Due to differences in altitude, brands of flour, etc you may need to cook for longer or shorter periods in time. Keep that in mind if yours are too doughy or crispy.)

Nutrition Info : Calories: 194kcal, Carbohydrates: 19g, Protein: 3g, Fat: 4g, Sodium: 24mg, Potassium: 76mg, Fiber: 5g

Air Fryer Pork Taquitos

Prep/Cook Time: 14 mins, 10 Servings, 8 W W Smart Points

Ingredients

- 3 cups cooked shredded pork tenderloin or chicken
- 2 1/2 cups fat free shredded mozzarella
- 10 small flour tortillas
- 1 lime, juiced
- Cooking spray

Instructions

- Preheat air fryer to 380 degrees.
- Sprinkle lime juice over pork and gently mix around.
- Microwave 5 tortillas at a time with a damp paper towel over it for 10 seconds, to soften.
- Add 3 oz. of pork and 1/4 cup of cheese to a tortilla.
- Tightly and gently roll up the tortillas.
- Line tortillas on a greased foil lined pan.
- Spray an even coat of cooking spray over tortillas.
- Air Fry for 7-10 minutes until tortillas are a golden color, flipping half way through.
- 2 taquitos per serving WW SP - 8.
- But in case you don't have an air fryer, they can also be baked in the oven for 7 - 10 minutes on 375 degrees.

Nutrition Info : Calories: 124kcal, Carbohydrates: 9g, Protein: 7g, Fat: 9g, Sodium:40mg, Fiber: 6g

Air Fryer Chimichangas

Prep/Cook Time: 34 minutes Servings : 8, 3 W W Smart Points

Ingredients

For the Chicken:

- 4 cups of deli-style cooked shredded rotisserie chicken or shredded chicken breast
- 1 large onion, finely chopped
- 1 4oz. can chopped green chilies
- 4 tbsp all-purpose flour
- 1 16 oz can of red enchilada sauce.
- ¼ tsp garlic powder
- 1 tsp ground cumin
- 8 (6 in) flour tortillas

Toppings for Chimichangas (optional)

- Reduced Fat Cheddar Cheese
- Plain Greek Yogurt
- Cilantro or Scallions

Instructions

- Preheat air fryer to 400°F. Coat a large skillet with cooking spray.
- Add onions and green chilies to pan and saute for 2 minutes. When the onions are soft add flour, salt, cumin, garlic powder, enchilada sauce, and continue stirring. When the sauce has thickened add in

precooked shredded chicken. If the sauce looks too thick add in some chicken stock to thin it out. (2 tablespoons to start)
- Take off heat and begin preparing the chimichangas for cooking them in the air fryer.
- Assemble chimichangas by spooning about 1/2 cup of chicken mixture onto each tortilla; fold in sides and roll up.
- Spray the outside of each filled tortilla with cooking spray; place 4 in the basket of air fryer, seam side down. Set to 400°F; cook 4 minutes. Turn; cook 2 to 3 minutes or until lightly browned and heated through. Repeat with remaining 4 filled tortillas.

Nutrition Info : Calories: 311, Sugar: 3, Sodium: 374, Fat: 7, Saturated Fat: 1, Carbohydrates: 20, Fiber: 2, Protein: 43

Weight Watchers Donuts

Prep/Cook Time: 20 minutes, 4 Servings, 3 W WSmart Points

Ingredients

- 1 cup nonfat Greek yogurt
- 1 cup self-rising flour, divided
- 1 tablespoon vanilla bean paste
- 1/2 cup cinnamon Splenda mixture
- optional: glaze (powdered sugar + water mixed)

Instructions

- Combine nonfat Greek yogurt plus 3/4 self-rising flour and 1 tablespoon vanilla bean paste.
- Roll out onto floured surface using the other 1/4 cup flour.
- Divide into 5 parts. Roll up to make donuts.

- Cook in air fryer at 375* for 4 minutes. Flip over and cook for another 3-4 minutes. (Due to differences in altitude, brands of flour, etc you may need to cook at 400 for up to 15 minutes. Keep that in mind if yours are doughy inside.)
- Spray with non-stick cooking spray, then dip in cinnamon and Splenda.
- Optional: drizzle with glaze.

Nutrition Info : Calories: 244, Sugar: 4, Fat: 8, Saturated Fat: 3, Carbohydrates: 18, Fiber: 3, Protein: 51

Air Fryer Funnel Cake Bites

Prep/Cook Time: 20 mins, 4 Servings, 3 W WSmart Points

Ingredients
- 1 cup nonfat Greek yogurt
- 1 cup self-rising flour, divided
- optional: 1 tablespoon vanilla bean paste
- powdered sugar for dusting

Instructions
- Combine nonfat Greek yogurt plus 3/4 self-rising flour and 1 tablespoon vanilla bean paste.
- Roll out onto floured surface using the other 1/4 cup flour.
- Cut into 32(ish) squares.
- Cook 8 at a time in Air Fryer at 375* for 4 minutes. Flip over and cook for another 3-4 minutes. (Due to differences in altitude, brands of flour, etc you may need to cook for longer or shorter periods in time. Keep that in mind if yours are too doughy or crispy.)
- Dust with powdered sugar while still warm.

Nutrition Info : 60 Cal, 80g Carbs, 44g Fat, 8g Protein

Air Fryer Tuna Cakes Recipe

Prep/Cook Time: 15 mins, Serves: 1, 3 W W Smart Points

Ingredients

- 1 3oz. can tuna in water
- 1 tablespoon flour
- 1 teaspoon light mayonnaise
- 1/8 teaspoon garlic powder
- 1/8 teaspoon dried dill
- 1/8 teaspoon salt
- 1/8 teaspoon black pepper

Instructions

- Drain water from tuna
- In a small bowl, mix all ingredients together until well blended. Will be slightly moist, but should be able to form patties.
- Divide into 4 equal portions, and create small circular patties.
- Lay in the basket of air fryer in a single layer.
- Following your air fryer Instructions, close and set to 380 degrees for 10 minutes. You may flip each patty halfway through if preferred, but it will cook well either way.

Nutrition Info : 325 calories; 15.5 g fat; 13.9 g carbohydrates; 31.3 g protein; 125 mg cholesterol; 409 mg sodium.

CONCLUSION

The weight watchers diet is appealing for a very good reason. It lets you eat what you want, within reason, as long as you don't eat too much of it. If you account for all your points, your weight loss plan will work wonders, and the pounds will melt away!